# Challenges in Older Women's Health

Heidi W. Brown • Makeba Williams
Sarina Schrager
Editors

# Challenges in Older Women's Health

## A Guide for Clinicians

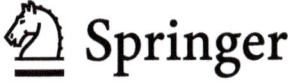

*Editors*
Heidi W. Brown
Division of Female Pelvic Medicine and
Reconstructive Surgery
Department of Obstetrics and Gynecology
University of Wisconsin
School of Medicine and Public Health
Madison, WI
USA

Makeba Williams
Division of Academic Specialists in
Obstetrics and Gynecology
Department of Obstetrics and Gynecology
University of Wisconsin
School of Medicine and Public Health
Madison, WI
USA

Sarina Schrager
Department of Family Medicine and
Community Health
University of Wisconsin
School of Medicine and Public Health
Madison, WI
USA

ISBN 978-3-030-59057-4     ISBN 978-3-030-59058-1  (eBook)
https://doi.org/10.1007/978-3-030-59058-1

© Springer Nature Switzerland AG 2021
This work is subject to copyright. All rights are reserved by the Publisher, whether the whole or part of the material is concerned, specifically the rights of translation, reprinting, reuse of illustrations, recitation, broadcasting, reproduction on microfilms or in any other physical way, and transmission or information storage and retrieval, electronic adaptation, computer software, or by similar or dissimilar methodology now known or hereafter developed.
The use of general descriptive names, registered names, trademarks, service marks, etc. in this publication does not imply, even in the absence of a specific statement, that such names are exempt from the relevant protective laws and regulations and therefore free for general use.
The publisher, the authors, and the editors are safe to assume that the advice and information in this book are believed to be true and accurate at the date of publication. Neither the publisher nor the authors or the editors give a warranty, expressed or implied, with respect to the material contained herein or for any errors or omissions that may have been made. The publisher remains neutral with regard to jurisdictional claims in published maps and institutional affiliations.

This Springer imprint is published by the registered company Springer Nature Switzerland AG
The registered company address is: Gewerbestrasse 11, 6330 Cham, Switzerland

*This book is dedicated to the older women who have touched our lives. We are grateful for your wisdom and strength.*

# Preface

The number of Americans over the age of 65 years is projected to more than double to over 98 million over the next 40 years. By 2060, this age group will comprise nearly 24 percent of the population. With an average life expectancy of 81, women can expect to live 30 years past menopause. Despite the growing population of older women, many clinicians who provide primary care receive minimal training about the unique health issues and needs of older women, and even fewer resources exist to guide practice.

*Challenges in Older Women's Health: A Primer for Clinicians* culls a diverse group of expert editors and authors to share a collection of chapters that serves as a practical tutorial for the care of older women's health needs. Our goal was to bring a multidisciplinary perspective that recognizes the need to eliminate disparate care in this vulnerable population and to help women discuss and tackle uncomfortable issues. Each chapter provides user-friendly, evidence-based guidance to manage common health challenges for women during menopause and beyond and provides resources for more in-depth study.

This book covers general topics such as menopause, bone health, cancer survivorship, and obesity. We specifically include topics often perceived as taboo or controversial, but critically important to older women's health, such as "Sexual Health and Function After Menopause," written by two obstetrician-gynecologists and a sex therapist, and "Bladder and Bowel Continence in Older Women," written by experts in Female Pelvic Medicine and Reconstructive Surgery. "Depression and Grief" provides an excellent overview of how to evaluate and manage these common conditions, including helpful tools to screen for elder abuse and tables of medications that are safest for use in older adults. "Breast Cancer Screening in Older Women" summarizes conflicting guidelines about screening for breast cancer across the life span and incorporates links to free interactive materials to guide shared decision-making.

While there is copious literature about the menopausal transition, almost no resources for clinicians exist about caring for women beyond the sixth decade. We hope that you find these chapters provide focused, high-yield, and evidence-based information about topics relevant to caring for our mothers and grandmothers: a too-often neglected group of patients.

Heidi W. Brown, MD, MAS, FACOG
Makeba Williams, MD, NCMP, FACOG
Sarina Schrager, MD, MS

# Acknowledgements

We would like to thank Dr. Laura Jacques and Dr. Rachel Kornik for graciously providing photos for this book.

# Contents

1. **Menopause Management** ........................................ 1
   Makeba Williams

2. **Breast Cancer Screening in Older Women** ..................... 15
   Laura Bozzuto

3. **Bone Health in Older Women** ................................. 25
   Thomas Hahn, Jensena Carlson, Adrienne Hampton,
   and Sarina Schrager

4. **Depression and Grief in Older Women** ........................ 45
   Julia Lubsen, Jillian Landeck, and Melissa Stiles

5. **Caring for Caregivers** ...................................... 61
   Kendra D. Sheppard

6. **Cancer Survivorship in Women 65 Years and Older** ............ 67
   James E. Haine, Noelle K. LoConte, and Amye J. Tevaarwerk

7. **Obesity and Aging** .......................................... 87
   Parvathi Perumareddi, Joanna Drowos, and Elizabeth Lownik

8. **Insomnia and Sleep Disorders in Older Women** ................ 105
   Krishna M. Desai, Heather L. Paladine, and Nataliya Pilipenko

9. **Pelvic Organ Prolapse** ...................................... 125
   Christina Escobar and Dominique Malacarne Pape

10. **Vulvar Pathology in Older Women** ........................... 145
    Emily R. Rosen

11. **Bladder and Bowel Continence in Older Women** ............... 163
    Heidi W. Brown, Candace Parker-Autry, and Angela L. Sergeant

12. **Sexual Health and Function in Menopause and Beyond** ........ 185
    Lauren Verrilli, Madelyn Esposito-Smith, and Makeba Williams

**Index** ......................................................... 201

# Contributors

**Laura Bozzuto, MD, MS, FACOG** Division of Academic Specialists in Obstetrics and Gynecology, Department of Obstetrics and Gynecology, Division of Surgical Oncology, Department of Surgery, University of Wisconsin School of Medicine and Public Health, Madison, WI, USA

**Heidi W. Brown, MD, MAS, FACOG** Division of Female Pelvic Medicine and Reconstructive Surgery, Department of Obstetrics and Gynecology, University of Wisconsin School of Medicine and Public Health, Madison, WI, USA

**Jensena Carlson, MD** Department of Family Medicine and Community Health, University of Wisconsin School of Medicine and Public Health, Madison, WI, USA

**Krishna M. Desai, MD, FAAFP** Center for Family and Community Medicine, Columbia University Irving Medical Center, New York, NY, USA

**Joanna Drowos, DO, MPH, MBA** Division of Family Medicine, Department of Integrated Medical Science Charles E Schmidt College of Medicine at Florida Atlantic University, Boca Raton, FL, USA

**Christina Escobar, MD, FACOG** Department of Obstetrics and Gynecology, New York University Medical Center, New York, NY, USA

**Madelyn Esposito-Smith, MA, LPC, NCC, CST** Department of Psychiatry, University of Wisconsin Medical Foundation, Madison, WI, USA

**Thomas Hahn, MD** Department of Family Medicine and Community Health, University of Wisconsin School of Medicine and Public Health, Madison, WI, USA

**James E. Haine, MD** Division of General Internal Medicine, Department of Internal Medicine, University of Wisconsin School of Medicine and Public Health, Madison, WI, USA

**Adrienne Hampton, MD** Department of Family Medicine and Community Health, University of Wisconsin School of Medicine and Public Health, Madison, WI, USA

**Jillian Landeck, MD** Department of Family Medicine and Community Health, University of Wisconsin School of Medicine and Public Health, Madison, WI, USA

**Noelle K. LoConte, MD** Department of Medicine, University of Wisconsin Carbone Cancer Center, University of Wisconsin School of Medicine and Public Health, Madison, WI, USA

**Elizabeth Lownik, MD, MPH** Department of Family Medicine and Community Health, University of Wisconsin School of Medicine and Public Health and Dean Medical Group/SSM Health, Madison, WI, USA

**Julia Lubsen, MD** Department of Family Medicine and Community Health, University of Wisconsin School of Medicine and Public Health, Madison, WI, USA

**Dominique Malacarne Pape, MD, FACOG** Department of Obstetrics and Gynecology, New York University Medical Center, New York, NY, USA

**Heather L. Paladine, MD, MEd, FAAFP** Center for Family and Community Medicine, Columbia University Irving Medical Center, New York, NY, USA

**Candace Parker-Autry, MD** Division of Female Pelvic Health, Department of Urology, Wake Forest Baptist Health, Winston-Salem, NC, USA

**Parvathi Perumareddi, DO** Charles E Schmidt College of Medicine at Florida Atlantic University, Boca Raton, FL, USA

**Nataliya Pilipenko, Ph.D., ABPP** Center for Family and Community Medicine, Columbia University Irving Medical Center, New York, NY, USA

**Emily R. Rosen, MD, FACOG** Department of Obstetrics and Gynecology, The Ohio State University, Columbus, OH, USA

**Sarina Schrager, MD, MS** Department of Family Medicine and Community Health, University of Wisconsin School of Medicine and Public Health, Madison, WI, USA

**Angela L. Sergeant, RN, ANP-BC** Division of Female Pelvic Medicine and Reconstructive Surgery, Department of Obstetrics and Gynecology, University of Wisconsin School of Medicine and Public Health, Madison, WI, USA

**Kendra D. Sheppard, MD, MSPH, CMD** Sheppard Consulting Services, LLC, Birmingham, AL, USA

**Melissa Stiles, MD** Department of Family Medicine and Community Health, University of Wisconsin School of Medicine and Public Health, Madison, WI, USA

**Amye J. Tevaarwerk, MD** Division of Hematology, Oncology and Palliative Care, Department of Medicine, University of Wisconsin Carbone Cancer Center, University of Wisconsin School of Medicine and Public Health, Madison, WI, USA

**Lauren Verrilli, MD** Division of Reproductive Endocrinology and Infertility, Department of Obstetrics and Gynecology, University of Utah School of Medicine, Salt Lake City, UT, USA

**Makeba Williams, MD, NCMP, FACOG** Division of Academic Specialists in Obstetrics and Gynecology, Department of Obstetrics and Gynecology, University of Wisconsin School of Medicine and Public Health, Madison, WI, USA

# Menopause Management

Makeba Williams

**Key Points**
1. Approximately 42% of women aged 60–65 will experience hot flashes and night sweats during menopause.
2. Approximately 50% of women will experience genitourinary syndrome of menopause (GSM): chronic, progressive genitourinary changes such as vulvovaginal dryness and atrophy, increased vaginal and urinary infections, as well as genitourinary discomfort and pain.
3. Hormonal and nonhormonal treatment options are available to treat older women in menopause.
4. Shared decision-making should be used to individualize treatment of symptomatic menopausal women.
5. Hormone therapy should not be used to prevent chronic disease, cancer, mood, or cognitive changes.

**Case**
Ann is a 57-year-old patient who presents with hot flashes and night sweats. She reports that menopause occurred at age 52, and she immediately began to experience bothersome hot flashes and night sweats. Her symptoms were relieved completely when her primary care provider prescribed combined

---

M. Williams (✉)
Division of Academic Specialists in Obstetrics and Gynecology,
Department of Obstetrics and Gynecology, University of Wisconsin School of Medicine and Public Health, Madison, WI, USA
e-mail: MWilliams28@wisc.edu

hormone therapy containing estrogen and progesterone. After 2 years of hormone therapy, her primary care provider discontinued the hormone therapy out of concern for an increased risk of cancer and cardiovascular disease. She now has had a return of symptoms: severe hot flashes, approximately five to ten per day, sleep disrupted by night sweats, and uncomfortable sex, which she attributes to an increasingly dry vagina. She has tried over-the-counter herbs and supplements to relieve her symptoms; they have not helped. Glycerin and water-based lubricants did not help her vaginal symptoms.

Menopause results from the permanent cessation of ovarian function secondary to natural senescence of the ovaries or iatrogenic disruption of ovarian function secondary to surgical removal or damage from chemotherapy or radiation. Natural menopause is diagnosed after the cessation of menses for 1 year, and is on average diagnosed at age 51 in the United States. With an average life expectancy of 81.6 years, women in the United States can expect to spend more than 30 years in menopause [1]. The decline in ovarian function and hormone production—estrogen, progesterone, and testosterone—leads to a number of physiologic changes during the menopausal transition. Women frequently complain of vasomotor symptoms (VMS), also known as hot flashes and night sweats, genitourinary symptoms such as vaginal dryness, as well as changes in memory, mood, sleep, and weight. Vasomotor complaints are the most commonly discussed symptoms of menopause. The etiology of these hot flashes is incompletely understood, but is thought to be related to dysregulation of the thermoneutral regulatory zone in the hypothalamus. Hot flashes are thought to occur when the core body temperature is triggered to rise above the upper threshold of this narrow thermoneutral zone; shivering occurs when the core body temperature falls below the lower threshold. Recent research has implicated the KNDy—kisspeptin, neurokinin B, and dynorphin— neuron complex located in the arcuate nucleus as a mediator of estrogen signals to the thermoregulatory center [2].

Vasomotor symptoms are characterized by intense, recurrent episodes of warmth that begin centrally and progress to the upper body, culminating in flushing of the face followed by chills and sweating; 75–80% of menopausal women will experience bothersome hot flashes that may occur during waking hours or sleep [3, 4].

When these symptoms occur at night, they are referred to as night sweats; they often occur during and are disruptive to sleep. Vasomotor symptoms can vary in severity and frequency.

While vasomotor symptoms appear to be most intense during the menopausal transitions and early menopausal periods, these symptoms may continue and adversely impact the quality of life of older women. Nearly 20% of women visiting a menopausal consultation clinic at the Mayo Clinic were 60 years of age or older [5].

Forty-two percent of women aged 60–65 will experience moderate to severe hot flashes [6]. About 12% of women aged greater than 67 and ~20 years beyond the age of menopause report clinically significant vasomotor symptoms [7]. 16% of Swedish women older than age 85 report vasomotor symptoms several times per

**Table 1.1** Conditions and medications that trigger or mimic vasomotor symptoms

*Tumors/cancer*: hypothalamic, pituitary gland, pheochromocytoma, carcinoid, pancreatic, renal cell
*Diet*: alcohol, spicy foods, monosodium glutamate (MSG)
*Infections*: tuberculosis or HIV
*Medical conditions*: thyroid disorder, mast cell disorders
*Medications*: chronic opioid use or opioid withdrawal, SSRIs, nitroglycerin, nifedipine, niacin, vancomycin, calcitonin, and antiestrogens (such as tamoxifen or aromatase inhibitors)
*Anxiety disorders*

week, though only 6% were using hormone therapy (HT) to treat these symptoms [8]. The presence of vasomotor symptoms has implications for poorer physical and psychological health: increased risk of coronary heart and cardiovascular disease, osteoporosis, and increased depression [9–11]. Women with hot flashes have increased visits for outpatient health care.

The costs, direct and indirect, associated with treating vasomotor symptoms is estimated to be hundreds of million dollars annually. Vasomotor symptoms are clinically diagnosed through patient report and history. Associated risks factors include: cigarette smoking, obesity, depressive symptoms, low educational attainment, and African American ethnicity [4, 12].

It is important to rule out other conditions as these symptoms can be provoked by medications, infections, endocrinopathies, and infections in older women (Table 1.1).

Laboratory measurement of hormone levels is often unnecessary to make a diagnosis of menopausal vasomotor symptoms. Women often report a sudden feeling of intense heat that begins centrally, radiates to the upper body and face, followed by increased sweating in the same areas. These hot flashes typically last about 2–5 min. The skin temperature may rise 1–7° and the heart rate may increase 5–7 beats/min. Following the resolution of the hot flash and sweating, women may also experience chills due to the rapid decline in skin and core body temperature.

## Treatment

Estrogen therapy is the most effective treatment of vasomotor symptoms. For women with intact uteri, progestogen therapy is required for endometrial protection from the proliferative effects of systemic estrogen on the endometrium. A Cochrane review showed that estrogen alone, or combined with progestogen, is significantly more effective than placebo in reducing the severity of vasomotor symptoms and the frequency of symptoms by 75% [13]. Unfortunately, there has been a marked decline in the use of hormone therapy since the release of the Women's Health Initiative (WHI) study results in 2002. This randomized control trial was designed to assess the benefits of hormone therapy for chronic disease prevention and cancer in a healthy menopausal cohort. Patients who received estrogen alone had reduction in breast cancer risk, no increase in cardiovascular disease events, and a decrease in risk of fractures and colon cancer. Five years of estrogen–progestogen use resulted in a nominal increased risk of coronary heart disease (CHD), breast cancer, venous thromboembolic disease, and strokes.

The majority of the study population were older than age 60 and the oldest participants aged 79 [14]. Very few women in the trial reflected the population for whom hormone therapy is typically prescribed, women who are within 10 years of the final menstrual period and less than 60 years of age. These results have been overgeneralized to women of all age ranges and hormone therapy formulations, despite utilizing one route of administration, oral, and one formulation of estrogen: conjugate equine estrogen (CEE) or medroxyprogesterone acetate (MPA). More recent hormone therapy trials and follow-up reanalysis of the WHI results provide additional perspectives and guidance about the safe use of hormone therapy to treat menopausal symptoms. Moreover, 18-year follow-up data from the WHI show that the use of CEE with MPA for 5.6 years or CEE alone for 7.2 years was not associated with an increased risk of all-cause, cardiovascular, or total cancer mortality [15].

Based upon the best available data, hormone therapy is safe to use for the treatment of moderate to severe vasomotor symptoms and the genitourinary syndrome of menopause (GSM). Hormone therapy, however, should not be used to prevent chronic disease.

*The Bottom Line on Hormone Therapy from the Women's Health Initiative and observational studies*:

- The benefits of hormone therapy exceed the risk in most women.
- For women younger than age 60 or who are within 10 years of menopause and without contraindications, hormone therapy has a favorable benefit–risk ratio when used to treat moderate to severe vasomotor symptoms.
- The benefit–risk ratio is less favorable for women who *initiate* hormone therapy more than ten years after onset of menopause or who are older than age 60 due to the increased age-related risk of coronary heart disease, stroke, venous thromboembolism, and dementia.
- In 18 years of follow-up data, hormone therapy with conjugate equine estrogen plus medroxyprogesterone acetate for ~5 years or with conjugate equine estrogen alone for ~7.2 years, was not associated with risk of all-cause, cardiovascular, or cancer mortality during a cumulative follow-up of 18 years.
- Annual evaluation of symptoms and documentation of persistent symptoms as well as the shared decision-making process should occur in the setting of extended duration of use for persistent vasomotor symptoms [15, 16].

Hormone therapy (HT) is available in various formulations—oral, transdermal, and vaginal—and dose preparations—standard and low dose—all of which may yield variable response. The risks of HT differ depending on type, dose, duration of use, route of administration, timing of initiation, and whether a progestogen is used.

**Table 1.2** Combined hormone therapy

| Product name(s) | Estrogen | Progestogen |
|---|---|---|
| Prempro | 0.625 mg conjugated estrogens | 2.5 or 5 mg medroxyprogesterone acetate |
| | 0.3 or 0.45 conjugated estrogens | 1.5 mg medroxyprogesterone acetate |
| Femhrt | 5 µg ethinyl estradiol | 1 mg norethindrone acetate |
| | 2.5 µg ethinyl estradiol | 0.5 mg norethindrone acetate |
| Activella | 1 mg 17β-estradiol | 0.5 mg norethindrone acetate |
| | 0.5 mg 17β-estradiol | 0.1 mg norethindrone acetate |
| Angeliq | 0.5 mg 17β-estradiol | 1 mg drospirenone |
| | 0.25 mg 17β-estradiol | 0.5 mg drospirenone |
| Climara Pro | 0.045 mg 17β-estradiol | 0.015 mg levonorgestrel |
| CombiPatch | 0.05 mg 17β-estradiol | 0.14 mg norethindrone acetate |
| Duavee | 0.45 mg conjugated estrogens + 20 mg bazedoxifene | |

Treatment should be individualized to identify the most appropriate HT type, dose, formulation, route of administration, and duration of use, using the best available evidence to maximize benefits and minimize risks, with periodic reevaluation of the benefits and risks for continuing or discontinuing HT. Individualization is likely to improve *symptom relief, optimize patient adherence and satisfaction, and minimize associated risks.*

Commonly prescribed hormonal therapies may be found in Tables 1.2, 1.3, and 1.4.

## Commonly Prescribed Hormone Therapies

A list of updated government-approved drugs for the treatment of menopausal symptoms may be found at http://www.menopause.org/docs/default-source/professional/nams-ht-tables.pdf [17]

*MenoPro* is a mobile app (https://www.menopause.org/for-professionals/-i-menopro-i-mobile-app) [18] produced by The North American Menopause Society (NAMS) that can be used by both clinicians and patients to individualize and personalize treatment decisions. It considers patients' personal treatment preferences, medical history, and underlying risk factors. Nonhormonal and hormonal treatment options are imbedded in the app.

Caution must be taken when considering the use of systemic hormone therapy to treat women more than 10 years from the diagnosis of menopause or those who are over the age of 60. Hormone therapy initiated between the age of 50 and 59, and within 10 years of the onset of menopause may be associated with a reduced risk of CHD [19]. However, initiating hormone therapy in women older than age 60 and in those women who are more than 10 years from the onset of menopause increases the risks of stroke, venous thromboembolism (VTE), and pulmonary embolism (PE) [20] for women who have age-related risks for these conditions. The NAMS,

**Table 1.3** Estrogen-only therapy

| Oral products | | |
|---|---|---|
| Composition | Product name(s) | Range of available dose strengths |
| Conjugated estrogens | Premarin | 0.3–1.25 mg |
| Synthetic conjugated estrogens, A | Cenestin | 0.3–1.25 mg |
| Synthetic conjugated estrogens, B | Enjuvia | 0.3–1.25 mg |
| Esterified estrogens | Menest | 0.3–1.25 mg |
| 17β-estradiol | Estrace, various generics | 0.5–2.0 mg |
| Estradiol acetate | Femtrace | 0.45–1.8 mg |
| Estropipate | Ortho-Est | 0.625 mg (0.75 mg estropipate, calculated as sodium estrone sulfate 0.625 mg) to 5.0 mg (6.0 mg) |
| Transdermal products | | |
| 17β-estradiol matrix patch | Alora, Climara, Esclim, Fempatch, Menostar, Vivelle, Vivelle-Dot, various generics | 0.014–0.1 mg delivered daily; applied once or twice weekly |
| 17β-estradiol reservoir patch | Estraderm | 0.05–0.1 mg delivered daily; applied twice weekly |
| 17β-estradiol transdermal gel | EstroGel, Elestrin, Divigel | Applied daily via metered pump or packet delivering 0.52–0.75 mg of 1/β-estradiol in gel |
| 17β-estradiol topical emulsion | Estrasorb | 2 packets applied daily |
| 17β-estradiol transdermal spray | Eva mist | 1 spray/d, up to 2–3/d if needed |
| Vaginal products | | |
| Estradiol acetate vaginal ring | Femring | Device containing 12.4 or 24.8 mg estradiol acetate releases 0.05 mg/d or 0.10 mg/d estradiol for 90 days (both doses release systemic levels for treatment of vulvovaginal atrophy and vasomotor symptoms) |

**Table 1.4** Progesterone only therapy

| Product name(s) | Composition | Dosage (mg/d) |
|---|---|---|
| Provera (generic(s) available) | Medroxyprogesterone acetate | 5, 10 (administer cyclically 12–14 d/mo) |
| Prometrium | Micronized progesterone | 200 (administer cyclically 12 d/28-d cycle) |
| *Levonorgestrel IUD** | *Levonorgestrel IUD* | *52 mg over a 5 year period* |

*Indicates off label use of the the Levonorgestrel IUD for endometrial protection

Endocrine Society, and American College of Obstetricians and Gynecologists (ACOG) advise against arbitrary age-related treatment discontinuation. Treatment decisions should be individualized through a shared decision-making framework that accounts for symptom severity, an analysis of risks and benefits of HT, and the patients' treatment goals. Annual evaluation of symptoms and treatment continuation is recommended [16, 21, 22].

For women who present with new onset vasomotor symptoms (VMS), it is important to evaluate for medications or other conditions that may contribute to VMS.

Systemic hormone therapy use is contraindicated in the setting of unexplained vaginal bleeding, severe active liver disease, prior estrogen-sensitive breast or endometrial cancer, coronary heart disease (CHD), stroke, dementia, personal history or inherited high risk of thromboembolic disease, porphyria cutanea tarda, or hypertriglyceridemia.

Many menopausal women report distressing sleep disruptions, mood instability, and cognitive impairment. All of the changes may be attributable to the general effects of aging. While these concerns should be fully evaluated, there is no clear benefit to using hormone therapy to treat sleep, mood, memory, dementia, or cognitive changes in women. Please see the chapters on sleep and depression for more guidance on evaluation and treatment.

> **Case (Continued)**
> Following a discussion of her symptoms and hormonal treatment options, Ann and her provider determine that she is a good candidate for hormone therapy; however, Ann wants to explore nonhormonal options as well.

For women who are not candidates for or elect to not use hormone therapy, there are many nonhormonal options. SSRIs and SNRIs are frequently used to treat vasomotor symptoms (Table 1.5). Paroxetine salt 7.5 mg is the only nonhormonal pharmacologic treatment approved by the FDA for moderate to severe vasomotor symptoms. The frequency and severity of vasomotor symptoms and sleep disruptions improve typically within 2 weeks, without increasing weight gain or diminishing libido. Off-label use of other SSRIs and SNRIs leads to mild to moderate improvement in VMS; these include escitalopram, citalopram, venlafaxine, desvenlafaxine, and paroxetine. Paroxetine and fluoxetine should be avoided in patients using tamoxifen as these drugs inhibit the CYP2D6 enzyme that converts tamoxifen to its active metabolite. SNRIs are safer, more effective options for these patients.

The gabapentinoids, gabapentin and pregabalin, are effective at improving hot flashes. Gabapentin may also improve sleep patterns in symptomatic patients. Suggested dosing for off-label use of gabapentin is 300 mg three times daily, 900 mg/day. Consider titrating slowly to reduce adverse side-effects such as dizziness, unsteadiness, and drowsiness. These side-effects typically improve in 1–2 weeks and resolve in 4 weeks.

Weight loss, mindfulness-based stress reduction, soy isoflavones derivatives and extracts, and stellate ganglion blockade are recommended with caution as there is evidence to suggest that these options may be beneficial in some circumstances; however, more evidence is needed. While lifestyle practices and modifications such

**Table 1.5** Suggested dosing ranges for nonhormonal prescription therapies

| SSRIs | | |
|---|---|---|
| Paroxetine salt | 7.5 mg | Single dose, no titration needed |
| Paroxetine | 10–25 mg/d | Start with 10 mg/d |
| Citalopram | 10–20 mg/d | Start with 10 mg/d |
| Escitalopram | 10–20 mg/d | Start with 10 mg/d (for sensitive or older women, start with 5 mg/d for titration, but this dose has not been tested for efficacy) |
| **SNRIs** | | |
| Desvenlafaxine | 100–150 mg/d | Start with 25–50 mg/d and titrate up by that amount each day |
| Venlafaxine | 37.5–150 mg/d | Start with 37.5 mg/d |
| **Gabapentinoids** | | |
| Gabapentin | 900–2,400 mg/d | Start with 300 mg at night, then add 300 mg at night, then a separate dose of 300 mg in the morning (start 100 mg if concerned about sensitivity) |
| Pregabalin | 150–300 mg/d | |

Abbreviations: *SNRIs* serotonin-norepinephrine reuptake inhibitors, *SSRIs* selective serotonin reuptake inhibitors

as exercise, yoga, cooling, and avoidance of triggers that may provoke vasomotor symptoms (spicy foods, alcohol, hot foods, or liquids) are reasonable and may be beneficial to overall health, there is good evidence that they are unlikely to alleviate quality of life. Herb and supplements, black cohosh, evening primrose oil, omega-3s, ginseng, vitamins, among other over-the-counter products, should not be recommended until higher-quality trials are performed that demonstrate their efficacy.

> **Case (Continued)**
> Prior to making a final decision about treating her vasomotor symptoms, Ann wishes to learn more about treatment for vaginal dryness and sexual discomfort.

## Genitourinary Syndrome of Menopause (GSM)

The lack of estrogen following menopause directly impacts the urogenital and vulvovaginal tissues. Estrogen receptors are highly concentrated in the urogenital tract along the bladder trigone, the vulvar, and vaginal tissues. The loss of estrogen then results in numerous physical changes to these tissues: decreased collagen, elastic and vascular flow, and increased alkalization of the vagina. The decreased estrogenic state results in thinning, inflammation, keratinization, and atrophy for the vulvovaginal tissue [23].

As the vaginal pH becomes more basic causing shifts in the vaginal flora, the risk for vaginal infections increases. The vulvovaginal tissue becomes less flexible and elastic. The labia minora and vaginal epithelium become thin and the vaginal rugae

**Table 1.6** Genitourinary syndrome of menopause: symptoms and signs

| |
|---|
| *Symptoms* |
|    Vulvar pain, burning, or itching |
|    Vaginal dryness or discharge |
|    Dyspareunia |
|    Spotting or bleeding after intercourse |
|    Urinary pain or discomfort, frequency, urgency, or recurrent infections |
| *Signs, external genitalia* |
|    Decreased labial size |
|    Loss of vulvar fat pads |
|    Vulvar fissures |
|    Receded or phimotic clitoris |
|    Prominent urethra with mucosal eversion or prolapse |
| *Signs, vagina* |
|    Introital narrowing |
|    Loss of elasticity with constriction |
|    Thin vaginal epithelial lining |
|    Loss of mature squamous epithelium |
|    Pale or erythematous appearance |
|    Petechiae, ulcerations, or tears |
|    Alkaline pH (>5.5) |
|    Infection (yellow or greenish discharge) |

Source: Adapted from Ref. [28]

diminish. The introital tissues retract leading to a more prominent urethra meatus, which is subject to increased irritation and trauma. Acute and recurrent urinary tract infections (UTIs) may become more prevalent [24].

Collectively, these changes (Table 1.6) are termed the genitourinary syndrome of menopause (GSM) and are experienced by as many as 50% of menopausal women [24–26].

Women may report vaginal dryness, burning, itching, and irritation; and urinary frequency, urgency, and dysuria. Patients may experience these symptoms in the absence of sexual activity; those who are sexually active may experience dyspareunia and postcoital bleeding due to decreased lubrication of the vagina and vulvar tissues. Many women report that these symptoms affect their quality of life. Despite the impact and prevalence of vulvovaginal symptoms, the GSM is often underdiagnosed and undertreated by many health care providers. Less than 5% of menopausal patients recognize these symptoms as being related to menopause [27].

## Treatments for Sexual Dysfunction Related to Genitourinary Syndrome of Menopause

Unlike vasomotor symptoms, GSM symptoms are chronic and progressive and do not improve over time unless they are treated, and will only get worse if not treated. First-line treatment for mild GSM includes *vaginal moisturizers and lubricants* (Table 1.7). Moisturizers do not cure atrophic conditions; however, using them two to three times weekly can provide temporary relief by reducing pain, itching, and

**Table 1.7** Commonly recommended lubricants and moisturizers

| |
|---|
| *Lubricants* |
| Water based |
|   Astroglide Liquid, Astroglide Gel, Liquid Astroglide |
|   Just Like Me, K-Y Jelly, Pre-Seed, Slippery Stuff, Liquid Silk |
| Silicone based |
|   Astroglide X, ID Millennium, K-Y Intrigue Pink, Pjur, Eros |
| *Moisturizers* |
| Replens, Me Again, Vagisil, Feminease, K-Y SILK-E, Luvena, Sliken Secret |

**Table 1.8** Nonpharmacologic therapies for GSM management

| |
|---|
| Education and normalization |
| Lubricants |
| Moisturizers |
| Painless stimulation or sexual activity |
| Vaginal dilators |
| Pelvic floor physical therapy |
| Psychotherapy/behavior counseling and/or sex therapy |

irritation [24]. Moisturizers containing hyaluronic acid have been found to normalize vaginal pH, reduce itching, dryness, dyspareunia, and improve symptoms of vaginal atrophy equivalent to local estrogen in some studies [29].

The options for over-the-counter lubricants and moisturizers are endless, though not all are created equally.

Many water-based lubricants have been found to be hyperosmolar with the potential to cause more damage to fragile vaginal tissue. The World Health Organization recommends lubricants not exceeding 380 mOsm/kg, though a maximum of 1200 mOSm/kg is acceptable. Recommended iso-osmolar products that fall within the pH range of a healthy vagina, 3.8–4.5, or those that are silicone based are ideal to prevent further tissue damage and recurrent UTIs, yeast infections, and bacterial vaginosis. Patients should avoid products containing flavors, warming properties, parabens, glycerin, and spermicides because they too may further irritate the vaginal and vulvar tissues. Natural oils (e.g., olive, coconut) may promote vaginal infections.

Vaginal dilators and pelvic floor physical therapy may be utilized to improve and maintain vaginal patency and caliber for women who experience vaginismus associated with decreased elasticity of the introitus and pelvic floor hypertonicity that may result in dyspareunia. (See also Chapter 12). A list of nonpharmacologic therapies for GSM management is provided in Table 1.8.

There are a number of pharmacologic treatment options for treating GSM (Table 1.9).

*Low-dose vaginal estrogen* is the most effective local treatment for GSM and is the preferred treatment option for sexual dysfunction related to genitourinary

**Table 1.9** Pharmacologic treatments for GSM

| Treatment | Product name(s) | Initial dose | Maintenance dose |
|---|---|---|---|
| *Vaginal products* | | | |
| *Creams* | | | |
| 17β-estradiol | Estrace Vaginal Cream | 0.5–1 gm/d for 2 wk | 0.5–1 gm/d × 1–3 per wk |
| Conjugated estrogens | Premarin Vaginal Cream | 0.5–1 gm/d for 2 wk | 0.5–1 gm 1–3 per wk |
| *Vaginal ring* | | | |
| 17β-estradiol vaginal ring | Estring | 2 mg releases 7.5 μg/d for 90 days | Change q 90d |
| *Vaginal inserts* | | | |
| Estradiol hemihydrate vaginal tablet | Vagifem, Yuvafem, generic | 10 μg insert 1/d × 2 wk | 1 tablet twice per wk |
| 17β-estradiol soft gel ovule | Imvexxy | 4 or 10 μg 1/d × 2 wk, followed by 1 ovule twice weekly | 1 gel ovule twice per wk |
| Prasterone (DHEA) | Intrarosa | 6.5 mg insert 1/d (DHEA) | 6.5 mg insert 1/d |
| *Vulvar products* | | | |
| Lidocaine | 4% Aqueous lidocaine | Applied to vestibule before sexual activity | |
| *Oral products* | | | |
| Ospemifene | Osphena | 60 mg/d orally | 60 mg/d orally |

symptoms of menopause. Estrogen is important for the maintenance and functioning of the vaginal epithelium, thickens the basalis layer, and plays an important role in vasodilation to increase vaginal, clitoral, and urethral blood flow [30].

Improvement in the vulvar and vaginal tissue may be seen within 6–8 weeks. Prior to the use of estrogen, a physical exam should be performed to confirm a hypoestrogenic state and to rule out other pathologies. Local vaginal estrogen is available in many forms: cream, tablet, soft gel ovule, vaginal ring. Most have similar efficacy; thus, patient preference, cost, and ease of administration should be discussed with patients when choosing a method.

Progesterone is not generally indicated for endometrial protection with the use of local estrogen, though safety data for >1 year are not available [16]. Long-term follow-up data are not available to provide guidance about the optimal duration of use of vaginal estrogen, especially in those women who are breast cancer survivors. Low-dose vaginal estrogen use for 1–18 years did not appear to be associated with changes in breast density or Bi-RADS breast cancer risk scores in a small cohort of women, which included three breast cancer survivors [31].

For women who simultaneously experience systemic vasomotor symptoms and GSM and vasomotor symptoms, *low-dose transdermal estradiol* has demonstrable benefit in increasing frequency of sexual activity, sexual fantasies, and degree of enjoyment, and causing decrease in pain during intercourse. However, arousal and orgasm were not enhanced by transdermal estradiol treatment [32].

*Ospemifene is a selective estrogen receptor modulator (SERM)* that has demonstrated statistical and clinical improvements in the vaginal maturation index, vaginal pH, and subjective vaginal dryness up to 1 year. With agonistic function at the genital tract and antagonistic properties on the breast and endometrial tissue, it has favorable effects on breast tissue and the endometrium, making it a safe option for current breast cancer patients or survivors or those in whom using an estrogen product is not ideal or desired. Clinical evidence shows decrease in palpable and abnormal mammographic findings, and the endometrium remains atrophic after 1 year of use [33].

In a review of preclinical and clinical studies, there were no reported cases of endometrial or breast cancer with ospemiphene use [34].

Ospemifene is dosed orally, 60 mg daily, and is a good option for those who cannot or prefer not to use a vaginal product. Patients may require a 6-month trial before noticing an improvement in dyspareunia. Ospemifene should be avoided in patients with undiagnosed vaginal bleeding, estrogen-dependent neoplasia, and inpatients with venous or arterial thromboembolic disease.

*Intravaginal dehydroepiandrosterone (DHEA), prasterone*, is FDA-approved for treatment of moderate to severe dyspareunia associated with GSM. Prasterone binds to both estrogen and androgen receptors and is aromatized to estrone and estradiol. Daily use is associated with clinically and statistically proven benefits in the vaginal maturation index, vaginal pH, vaginal dryness, and dyspareunia. While estrogen therapy is effective in the superficial mucosal layer, DHEA improves all three layers of the vaginal epithelium, improving the density of collagen fibers in the intermediate layer and stimulating the muscular third layer. Maximal benefits are seen after 2 weeks of daily dosing.

Currently, *no hormonal formulation has been FDA-approved for use in women with a history of hormone receptor positive breast cancer*. Nonhormonal therapy is first-line therapy for GSM symptoms in estrogen-sensitive breast and gynecologic cancer survivors. Prasterone, an estrogen precursor, has not yet been studied with breast cancer population. Use of vaginal estrogen or prasterone is considered off label and should be used with caution in estrogen- sensitive cancer survivors. The American Society of Clinical Oncology (ASCO) Sexual Health Guideline advises that clinicians may offer prasterone for women with a current or history of breast cancer who are on aromatase inhibitors and have not responded to previous treatment [35].

Use of estrogen and other hormone therapy in this population requires shared decision-making. Treatment should focus on the lowest effective dose for the least amount of time to enable function and alleviate symptoms [36]. The patient's oncology team should be consulted prior to initiating hormone therapy. Ospemifene use in breast cancer survivors is considered off label. While initial studies show promise in using $CO_2$ laser therapy therapy to improve GSM symptoms, the FDA has issued a warning against its use for these symptoms until further studies are conducted.

Numerous effective pharmacologic and nonpharmacologic options are available to treat both menopausal vasomotor and genitourinary symptoms for older women.

These include hormonal and nonhormonal treatment options. Shared decision-making and individualization are important to address the menopausal concerns of older women.

## References

1. Arias E, Xu J. United States life tables, 2017. Natl Vital Stat Rep. 2019;68(7):1–66.
2. Rance NE, Dacks PA, Mittelman-Smith MA, Romanovsky AA, Krajewski-Hall SJ. Modulation of body temperature and LH secretion by hypothalamic KNDy (kisspeptin, neurokinin B and dynorphin) neurons: a novel hypothesis on the mechanism of hot flushes. Front Neuroendocrinol. 2013;34(3):211–27.
3. Woods NF, Mitchell ES. Symptoms during the perimenopause: prevalence, severity, trajectory, and significance in women's lives. Am J Med. 2005;118(Suppl 12B):14–24.
4. Gold EB, Colvin A, Avis N, Bromberger J, Greendale GA, Powell L, et al. Longitudinal analysis of the association between vasomotor symptoms and race/ethnicity across the menopausal transition: study of women's health across the nation. Am J Public Health. 2006;96(7):1226–35.
5. David PS, Kling JM, Vegunta S, Faubion SS, Kapoor E, Mara KC, et al. Vasomotor symptoms in women over 60: results from the Data Registry on Experiences of Aging, Menopause, and Sexuality (DREAMS). Menopause. 2018;25(10):1105–9.
6. Gartoulla P, Worsley R, Bell RJ, Davis SR. Moderate to severe vasomotor and sexual symptoms remain problematic for women aged 60 to 65 years. Menopause. 2018;25(11):1331–8.
7. Huang AJ, Grady D, Jacoby VL, Blackwell TL, Bauer DC, Sawaya GF. Persistent hot flushes in older postmenopausal women. Arch Intern Med. 2008;168(8):840–6.
8. Vikström J, Spetz Holm AC, Sydsjö G, Marcusson J, Wressle E, Hammar M. Hot flushes still occur in a population of 85-year-old Swedish women. Climacteric. 2013;16(4):453–9.
9. Avis NE, Colvin A, Bromberger JT, Hess R, Matthews KA, Ory M, et al. Change in health-related quality of life over the menopausal transition in a multiethnic cohort of middle-aged women: Study of Women's Health across the Nation. Menopause. 2009;16(5):860–9.
10. Gast GC, Grobbee DE, Pop VJ, Keyzer JJ, Wijnands-van Gent CJ, Samsioe GN, et al. Menopausal complaints are associated with cardiovascular risk factors. Hypertension. 2008;51(6):1492–8.
11. Thurston RC, Sutton-Tyrrell K, Everson-Rose SA, Hess R, Matthews KA. Hot flashes and subclinical cardiovascular disease: findings from the study of Women's Health across the Nation Heart Study. Circulation. 2008;118(12):1234–40.
12. Gallicchio L, Miller SR, Kiefer J, Greene T, Zacur HA, Flaws JA. Risk factors for hot flashes among women undergoing the menopausal transition: baseline results from the Midlife Women's Health Study. Menopause. 2015;22(10):1098–107.
13. MacLennan A, Lester S, Moore V. Oral oestrogen replacement therapy versus placebo for hot flushes. Cochrane Database Syst Rev. 2001;1:CD002978.
14. Rossouw JE, Anderson GL, Prentice RL, LaCroix AZ, Kooperberg C, Stefanick ML, et al. Risks and benefits of estrogen plus progestin in healthy postmenopausal women: principal results from the Women's Health Initiative randomized controlled trial. JAMA. 2002;288(3):321–33.
15. Manson JE, Aragaki AK, Rossouw JE, Anderson GL, Prentice RL, LaCroix AZ, et al. Menopausal hormone therapy and long-term all-cause and cause-specific mortality: the Women's Health Initiative Randomized Trials. JAMA. 2017;318(10):927–38.
16. The 2017 hormone therapy position statement of the North American Menopause Society. Menopause 2018;25(11):1362–87.
17. Society TNAM. Approved prescription products for Menopausal symptoms in the United States and Canada. In: nams-ht-tables.pdf, editor. menopause.org: The North American Menopause Society; 2016.

18. Clinix D. MenoPro. In: Society TNAM, editor. 2014.
19. Manson JE, Allison MA, Rossouw JE, Carr JJ, Langer RD, Hsia J, et al. Estrogen therapy and coronary-artery calcification. N Engl J Med. 2007;356(25):2591–602.
20. Boardman HM, Hartley L, Eisinga A, Main C, Roqué i Figuls M, Bonfill Cosp X, et al. Hormone therapy for preventing cardiovascular disease in post-menopausal women. Cochrane Database Syst Rev. 2015;3:CD002229.
21. Stuenkel CA, Davis SR, Gompel A, Lumsden MA, Murad MH, Pinkerton JV, et al. Treatment of symptoms of the menopause: an endocrine society clinical practice guideline. J Clin Endocrinol Metab. 2015;100(11):3975–4011.
22. American College of Obstetricians and Gynecologists. Practice Bulletin No. 141. Management of menopausal symptoms: correction. Obstet Gynecol. 2018;131(3):604.
23. Goldstein I, Dicks B, Kim NN, Hartzell R. Multidisciplinary overview of vaginal atrophy and associated genitourinary symptoms in postmenopausal women. Sex Med. 2013;1(2):44–53.
24. Management of symptomatic vulvovaginal atrophy: 2013 position statement of the North American Menopause Society. Menopause. 2013;20(9):888–902; quiz 3–4.
25. MacBride M, Rhodes D, Shuster L. Vulvovaginal atrophy. Mayo Clin Proc. 2010;85:87–94.
26. Parish SJ, Nappi RE, Krychman ML, Kellogg-Spadt S, Simon JA, Goldstein JA, et al. Impact of vulvovaginal health on postmenopausal women: a review of surveys on symptoms of vulvovaginal atrophy. Int J Women's Health. 2013;5:437–47.
27. Nappi RE, Kokot-Kierepa M. Vaginal Health: Insights, Views & Attitudes (VIVA) - results from an international survey. Climacteric. 2012;15(1):36–44.
28. Portman DJ, Gass ML, Panel VATCC. Genitourinary syndrome of menopause: new terminology for vulvovaginal atrophy from the International Society for the Study of Women's Sexual Health and the North American Menopause Society. Menopause. 2014;21(10):1063–8.
29. Jokar A, Davari T, Asadi N, Ahmadi F, Foruhari S. Comparison of the hyaluronic acid vaginal cream and conjugated estrogen used in treatment of vaginal atrophy of menopause women: a randomized controlled clinical trial. Int J Community Based Nurs Midwifery. 2016;4(1):69–78.
30. Al-Azzawi F, Bitzer J, Brandenburg U, Castelo-Branco C, Graziottin A, Kenemans P, et al. Therapeutic options for postmenopausal female sexual dysfunction. Climacteric. 2010;13(2):103–20.
31. Zuo SW, Wu H, Shen W. Vaginal estrogen and mammogram results: case series and review of literature on treatment of genitourinary syndrome of menopause (GSM) in breast cancer survivors. Menopause. 2018;25(7):828–36.
32. Nathorst-Böös J, Wiklund I, Mattsson LA, Sandin K, von Schoultz B. Is sexual life influenced by transdermal estrogen therapy? A double blind placebo controlled study in postmenopausal women. Acta Obstet Gynecol Scand. 1993;72(8):656–60.
33. Palacios S, Cancelo MJ. Clinical update on the use of ospemifene in the treatment of severe symptomatic vulvar and vaginal atrophy. Int J Women's Health. 2016;8:617–26.
34. Archer DF, Simon JA, Portman DJ, Goldstein SR, Goldstein I. Ospemifene for the treatment of menopausal vaginal dryness, a symptom of the genitourinary syndrome of menopause. Expert Rev Endocrinol Metab. 2019;14(5):301–14.
35. Sussman TA, Kruse ML, Thacker HL, Abraham J. Managing genitourinary syndrome of menopause in breast cancer survivors receiving endocrine therapy. J Oncol Pract. 2019;15(7):363–70.
36. Farrell R, Practice ACoOaGCoG. ACOG committee Opinion No. 659: the use of vaginal estrogen in women with a history of estrogen-dependent breast cancer. Obstet Gynecol. 2016;127(3):e93–6.

# Breast Cancer Screening in Older Women

**2**

Laura Bozzuto

**Key Points**
- Randomized trials have consistently shown that screening mammography decreases breast cancer mortality in women aged 50–74.
- No randomized trials of breast cancer screening have included women over age 74.
- Women with less than 10 years of life expectancy likely will not benefit from screening detection of breast cancer.
- The majority of breast cancer risk for older women comes from age rather than hormonal exposures earlier in life.
- The decision to continue screening beyond age 74 should consider comorbidities and life expectancy, patient values, harms of screening, and the limited evidence in older women.

**Case**
Ms. Jones is a 77-year-old woman with hypertension, osteoarthritis, and obesity (BMI 37) who comes to clinic for her annual exam. She had a myocardial infarction with stent placement 2 years ago but lives independently. She went through menopause at age 50, had two children, the first at age 23, and has not

---

L. Bozzuto (✉)
Division of Academic Specialists in Obstetrics and Gynecology, Department of Obstetrics and Gynecology, Division of Surgical Oncology, Department of Surgery,
University of Wisconsin School of Medicine and Public Health, Madison, WI, USA
e-mail: bozzuto@wisc.edu

© Springer Nature Switzerland AG 2021
H. W. Brown et al. (eds.), *Challenges in Older Women's Health*,
https://doi.org/10.1007/978-3-030-59058-1_2

taken any hormone replacement therapy. She is engaged with her retired living community. She has continued to receive screening mammograms regularly since age 45. She had one breast biopsy at age 47 for calcifications that was benign. She wonders if she is due for a mammogram today.

## Breast Cancer Epidemiology

Breast cancer is the most common cancer for women in the United States, with approximately 12.8% of women being diagnosed with breast cancer in their lifetime [1]. The median age of diagnosis of breast cancer is 62 years. A significant proportion of women is diagnosed at older ages, with 31% of breast cancer diagnoses and 47% of breast cancer deaths in women 70 and older (Fig. 2.1) [1]. Breast cancer incidence increases with age and peaks at 452 cases per 100,000 women aged 70–79 [1, 2]. A woman in the USA who has remained cancer free to age 75 still has a 5.2% chance of developing breast cancer in her lifetime [3].

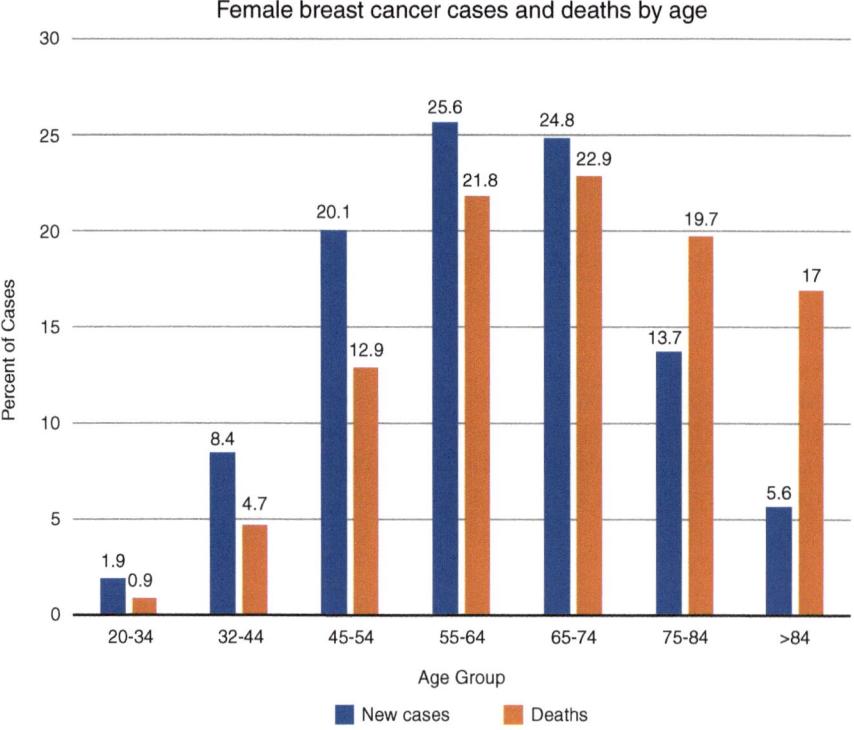

**Fig. 2.1** The chart displays the percentage of new breast cancer cases and breast cancer deaths by age group using data from the Surveillance, Epidemiology, and End Results (SEER) Program [1]. (Link: https://seer.cancer.gov/statfacts/html/breast.html)

## Screening Modalities

As with any screening program or test, the goals of breast cancer screening are to detect preclinical disease in asymptomatic patients, prevent adverse outcomes from more advanced stage at diagnosis, improve survival from detection at early stage, and decrease the need for more intense treatment.

## Mammography

Mammography is the gold standard for screening detection of breast cancer. Mammography has traditionally been performed in two views. In tomosynthesis, or 3D mammography, the X-ray tube is moved through an arc and images are reconstructed in layers [4]. This technology has been shown to have better ability to distinguish abnormalities in overlapping or dense breast tissue, which is less common in older patients.

The performance of mammography as a test to detect cancer increases with the age of patients. The sensitivity and specificity of mammography are highest in women over 80 (Table 2.1), leading to fewer false positive tests in this population [2].

## Clinical Breast Exams

Clinical breast exams (CBEs) may be offered to women, but there is uncertainty about the benefits (Table 2.2). A helpful video about CBE can be found at this link: https://www.youtube.com/watch?v=pJ55UtP0_nA

Table 2.1 Performance of screening mammography by age

|  | Sensitivity | Specificity | Positive predictive value |
|---|---|---|---|
| Age 50 | 73% | 92% | 22% |
| Age 80 | 86% | 94% | 41% |

Note: Table created using data from Walter et al. [2]

Table 2.2 Clinical breast exam recommendations for average-risk women by organization

|  | National Comprehensive Cancer Network [5] | American Cancer Society [6] | US Preventative Services Task Force [7] | American College of Obstetricians and Gynecologists [8] |
|---|---|---|---|---|
| Recommendation | Every 1–3 years for age 25–39; annually for age 40+ | Not recommended | Insufficient evidence to recommend for or against | May be offered in context of shared decision-making every 1–3 years for age 25–39; annually for age 40+ |

Systematic reviews conclude that clinical breast exams in addition to mammography increase detection of invasive cancers by 2–6% compared to mammogram alone, but also significantly increase the rate of false positives, and do not significantly improve outcomes [9, 10]. However, this research has been done in younger women, often simultaneously undergoing mammography. For older women, clinical breast exams may be an acceptable alternative after cessation of imaging screening.

## Other Screening Methods

Ultrasound and magnetic resonance imaging (MRI) are not recommended for primary screening for breast cancer. Ultrasound has been shown to have high false positives, is time intensive, and difficult to reproduce [11, 12]. MRI has high sensitivity but low specificity, and it is used as an adjunct screening method for high-risk patients. High-risk patients are defined as those with a BRCA 1 or 2 mutation, other known gene mutation conferring a high lifetime risk of breast cancer, history of mantle irradiation, or lifetime risk of breast cancer over 20% based on other factors like family history, prior atypia, or other exposures [5]. There are no guidelines on when to stop supplemental MRI screening for high-risk patients.

> **Case (Continued)**
> You explain to Ms. Jones that guidelines about screening mammography differ. While it is clear that screening mammography saves lives in women up to age 74, there are limited data to guide screening for women her age. She is terrified of breast cancer because her sister-in-law died from it. She feels like she is pretty healthy, other than knowing she should lose weight, and she would feel better continuing with annual mammograms. You order her mammogram.

## Estimating Benefits and Harms of Screening

### Benefits

Meta-analyses of randomized trials have consistently shown benefit from screening mammography in women aged 50–74, with decreases in breast cancer mortality of 15–25% for women in this age group [2, 7, 13, 14].

None of the prospective randomized trials have included women aged 75 or older. Retrospective cohort studies and case-control studies have shown reduction in breast cancer mortality with screening for older women in good health (Charlson comorbidity score < 2) [2]. Additionally, these studies show patients are diagnosed at earlier stages of disease, which may enable treatment with less aggressive options [3]. In one study, mammographic detection compared to physical exam detection of breast cancer was associated with a 50% lower risk of death in women 80 and older in good health [15]. These studies are at significant risk of selection and lead-time bias [2].

Cost-effectiveness analyses also show it is cost-effective to screen women biennially up until a life expectancy of 9.5 years [2, 16].

## Harms

Harms of breast cancer screening include pain, anxiety, cost, false positives, and overdiagnosis.

False positives are a significant risk for older women and lead to unnecessary tests and procedures with risks of complications. Among women 75 and older undergoing biennial screening, the cumulative probability over 10 years of screening of a false positive is 14–27%, a rate that doubles if annual screening is performed [2].

Cancers found by overdiagnosis are defined as cancer found by screening that would otherwise not affect the woman's overall health and lifespan if not detected [17]. This risk increases with age as life expectancy declines and with less aggressive cancers found in older women. Estimations of overdiagnosis of breast cancer range greatly, from 0 to 54%; however, most experts suggest a reasonable estimation at 30% [2].

## Guidelines

Differences in judgments about the balance of the benefits and harms of the evidence have led to lack of consensus among professional societies as to the ages to start and stop breast cancer screening, as well as the frequency of screening. Figure 2.2 displays breast screening recommendations by organization and includes recommendations from the American Cancer Society (ACS), the American College of Obstetricians and Gynecologists (ACOG), the American College of Radiologists (ACR), the United States Preventative Services Task Force (USPSTF), and the National Comprehensive Cancer Network (NCCN). Specific recommendations from each organization are listed in the caption.

Guidelines are limited in recommendations for older women. Because women 75 years and older were excluded from randomized controlled trials on breast cancer screening, there is limited evidence on which to base guideline recommendations. Because of the lack of trial data in older women, most guideline organizations recommend an individualized approach rather than a specific age cutoff (Table 2.3).

> **Case (Continued)**
> Ms. Jones' screening mammogram comes back with a new asymmetry in her left breast. She undergoes diagnostic mammogram and ultrasound, followed by a stereotactic biopsy. She develops a moderate hematoma after the biopsy. The results show a 7 mm grade 1 invasive ductal carcinoma that is estrogen receptor positive, progesterone receptor positive, and HER2 not amplified. She undergoes lumpectomy and sentinel node biopsy with a positive margin and requires a second surgical procedure. She then undergoes radiation. She has started an aromatase inhibitor for 5 years but now experiences significant joint pain and finds it difficult to remain as active as she once was.

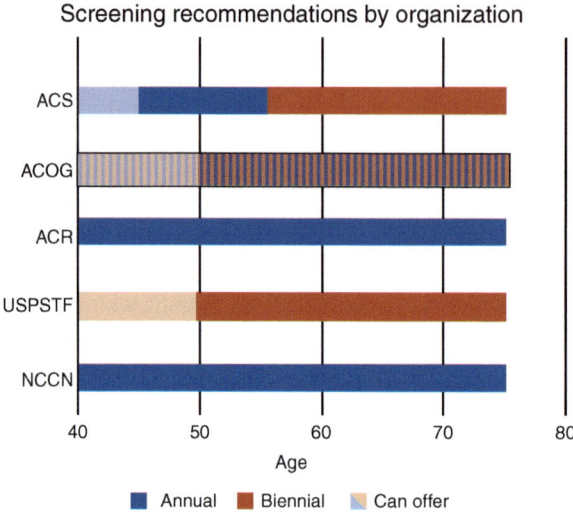

**Fig. 2.2** ACS: American Cancer Society [6, 9]; can offer age 40–45; recommend starting age 45; annual screening 40–54 if undertaken; biennial recommended after 54, but can continue annual. ACOG: American College of Obstetricians and Gynecologists [8]; screening age 40–49 after shared decision-making; recommend by age 50, annual or biennial. ACR: American College of Radiologists [18]; start age 40; annual. USPSTF: U.S. Preventative Services Task Force [7]; age 40–49; individual discussion; recommend starting age 50, biennial. NCCN: National Comprehensive Cancer Network [5]; start age 40; annual

**Table 2.3** Guidelines for screening mammography in older women

| Organization | Year issued | Screening recommendation |
|---|---|---|
| American Cancer Society [6] | 2015 | Screening should continue as long as a woman is in good health and is expected to live an additional 10 years or longer |
| American College of Obstetricians and Gynecologists [8] | 2017 | Continue until age 75 years; beyond age 75 years, the decision to discontinue should be based on a shared decision-making process that includes a discussion of the woman's health status and longevity |
| American College of Radiology [18] | 2017 | No recommendation to stop on basis of age; screening should be tailored to individual circumstances such as life expectancy, comorbidities, and intention to see and tolerate treatment; if performed, annual screening recommended |
| U.S. Preventative Services Task Force [7] | 2016 | No recommendation; evidence on mammography screening in women aged 75 and older is insufficient, and the balance of benefits and harms cannot be determined; (Cat I) |
| National Comprehensive Cancer Network [5] | 2019 | No established upper age limit for screening; if a patient has severe comorbid conditions limiting life expectancy and no further intervention would occur based on screening findings, then the patient should not undergo screening regardless of age |

## Estimating Breast Cancer Risk

In older women, age is the major risk factor for breast cancer [2]. Hormonal exposures in the distant past are less predictive of breast cancer risk in older women, and models that include these factors, such as the Gail model, perform poorly in women over 70 [2] (Link to Gail Model: https://bcrisktool.cancer.gov/calculator.html). One assessment of Gail model performance in a population of women 70 and older showed it accurately predicted breast cancer only 54% of the time [19].

## Breast Cancer Survivors

Some older women may have a distant history of breast cancer and no longer be followed by an oncologist. After a diagnosis of breast cancer, current guidelines from the American Cancer Society and American Society of Clinical Oncology (ASCO) recommend continued annual surveillance mammography for women with residual breast tissue due to evidence that recurrent or contralateral cancer events do not plateau [20]. However, this fails to take into consideration overall health status and the evidence that most older breast cancer survivors will die of other causes. More information about managing these patients can be found in Chapter 6.

A reasonable approach advocated by Freedman and others is to cease rigorous surveillance for women over 80 years or for women at any age with significant comorbidities and a life expectancy less than 5–10 years. Decisions can be individualized taking into consideration patient preferences and individual risk due to tumor biology and current treatment [20].

## Life Expectancy

Life expectancy should be considered when determining whether to stop or continue screening. Older women with three or more comorbidities are 20 times more likely to die of another cause than of breast cancer [3, 21].

A useful tool that incorporates age, comorbidities, and functional status to estimate life expectancy has been developed and validated and is available at the ePrognosis website [22] (link: eprognosis.ucsf.edu). Use of this tool provides both a risk of mortality over 1-, 5-, 10-, and 14-year time frames, and a median life expectancy given the patient's prognostic factors.

## Individualizing Screening

Discussing decisions about screening can be difficult for providers and patients. Older patients consistently overestimate the benefits of screening and underestimate the harms [2]. In a study from 2010, 56% of US women who were 75 years or older reported a screening mammogram in the prior 2 years, including 36% of women with a life expectancy less than 5 years [23].

Discussing the increasing harms of screening with age compared to decreasing benefits may be the most acceptable way to frame the discussion with patients. These include the harms of false positive tests, unnecessary biopsies, overdiagnosis, and lack of mortality benefit.

Additionally, patients and providers should consider the consequences of a positive screening test, including the ability for women to accept and tolerate the diagnostic workup and treatments for breast cancer, if detected.

One model of clinical decision-making for screening is presented in Fig. 2.3. Use of a shared decision-making model is recommended to discuss this choice. The patient's preferred role in decision-making should be assessed, along with her values. Clinical health information should be incorporated by the health provider in the conversation to individualize the discussion. Consideration of life expectancy should be included.

A useful online tool is available to guide this decision-making by integrating key health questions at ePrognosis for breast cancer screening. This tool generates a tailored risk assessment about whether screening is likely to help or harm this particular patient. The tool describes the risk of harm from screening, the risk of death from breast cancer, and the risk of death regardless of testing for breast cancer. This website also has useful communication resources to aid such conversations.

---

**Discussing Screening**

Doctor: Now that you are over 75, we should talk about your screening options for breast cancer.

Patient: Oh, I figured I would just keep getting mammograms.

Doctor: Well that is an option, but there is really not a lot of evidence for mammograms in older women and so we should be thoughtful about the potential harms and benefits for you. You do have some other health conditions that may affect your health more. For a woman your age in your health, only 1 out of 1000 would avoid death from breast cancer in the next 10 years, but 100 out of 1000 may experience an unnecessary biopsy or need treatment for a cancer that would never affect your life. Unfortunately, in the next 10 years 300 out of 1000 people like you would die regardless of if they were screened for breast cancer. What are your thoughts about this?

Patient: Are there any other options for screening?

Doctor: We should continue to do breast exams in the office. And we can continue to reassess this decision each year.

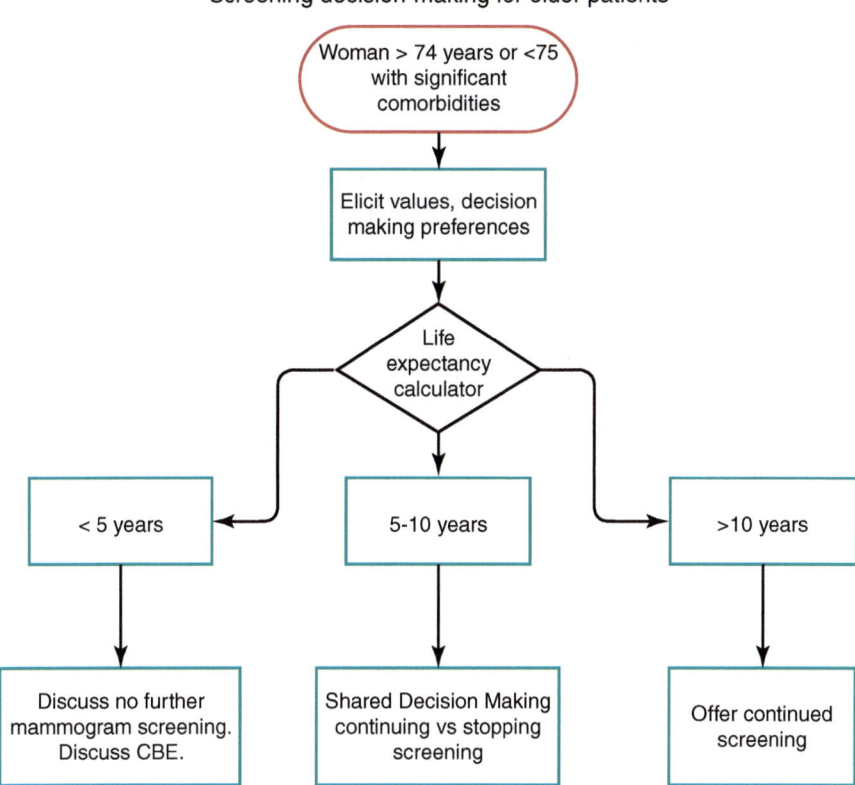

**Fig. 2.3** Use an assessment of life expectancy such as ePrognosis or Charlson comorbidity score. CBE: clinical breast exam. Link ePrognosis: https://eprognosis.ucsf.edu/. Link Charlson comorbidity score: https://www.mdcalc.com/charlson-comorbidity-index-cci

## Concluding Summary

Recommendations on breast cancer screening in older women are limited by the lack of studies performed in this population. Providers should keep in mind the length of time needed to benefit from screening and competing comorbidities when discussing these decisions with patients using a shared decision-making approach.

## References

1. SEER cancer stat facts: female breast cancer. Bethesda: National Cancer Institute. https://seer.cancer.gov/statfacts/html/breast.html
2. Walter LC, Schonberg MA. Screening mammography in older women: a review. JAMA. 2014;311(13):1336–47.
3. Lee CS, Moy L, Joe BN, Sickles EA, Niell BL. Screening for breast cancer in women age 75 years and older. AJR Am J Roentgenol. 2018;210:256–63.
4. Funaro K, Drukteinis J, Falcon S. Screening mammography and digital breast tomosynthesis: controversies. South Med J. 2017;110:607–13.
5. NCCN (National Comprehensive Cancer Network). Breast cancer screening and diagnosis. 2019;1.2019.
6. Michaelson JS, Shih YT, Walter LC, et al. Guideline update from the American Cancer Society. JAMA. 2016;314(15):1599–614.
7. Siu AL, on behalf of the USPSTF. Screening for breast cancer: U.S. preventative services task force recommendation statement. Ann Intern Med. 2016;164:279–96.
8. Cancer B, Assessment R. Practice bulletin no. 179 summary: breast cancer risk assessment and screening in average-risk women. Obstet Gynecol. 2017;130(1):241–3.
9. Oeffinger KC, Fontham ETH, Etzioni R, et al. Breast cancer screening for women at average risk: 2015 guideline update from the American Cancer Society. JAMA [Internet]. 2015;314(15):1599–614. Available from: https://doi.org/10.1001/jama.2015.12783.
10. Myers ER, Moorman P, Gierisch JM, et al. Benefits and harms of breast cancer screening: a systematic review. JAMA [Internet]. 2015;314(15):1615–34. Available from: https://doi.org/10.1001/jama.2015.13183.
11. Berg W, Zhang Z, Lehrer D, al et. Detection of breast cancer with addition of annual screening ultrasound or a single screening MRI to mammography in women with elevated breast cancer risk. JAMA 2012;307:1394–1404.
12. Lee C, Bassett L, Lehman C. Breast density legislation and opportunities for patient-centered outcomes research. Radiology. 2012;264:632–6.
13. Gotzche P, Jorgensen K. Screening for breast cancer with mammography (review). Cochrane Database Syst Rev. 2013;6:CD001877.
14. Independent UK panel on breast cancer screening. The benefits and harms of breast cancer screening: an independent review. Lancet. 2012;380:1778–86.
15. McPherson C, Swenson K, Lee M. The effects of mammographic detection and comorbidity on the survival of older women with breast cancer. J Am Geriatr Soc. 2002;50:1061–8.
16. Mandelblatt JS, Schechter CB, Yabroff KR, et al. Toward optimal screening strategies for older women. J Gen Intern Med. 2005;20:487–96.
17. Welch H, Black W. Overdiagnosis in cancer. J Natl Cancer Inst. 2010;102(9):605–13.
18. Monticciolo DL, Newell MS, Hendrick RE, et al. Breast cancer screening for average-risk women: recommendations from the ACR commission on breast imaging. J Am Coll Radiol [Internet]. 2019;14(9):1137–43. Available from: https://doi.org/10.1016/j.jacr.2017.06.001.
19. Vacek P, Skelly J, Geller B. Breast cancer risk assessment in women aged 70 and older. Breast Cancer Res Treat. 2011;130:291–9.
20. Freedman RA, Keating NL, Partridge AH, Muss HB, Hurria A, Winer EP. Mammography in older breast cancer survivors: can we ever stop? JAMA Oncol. 2017;3:402–9.
21. Satariano W, Ragland D. The effect of comorbidity on 3-year survival in women with primary breast cancer. Ann Intern Med. 1994;120:104–10.
22. Yourman L, Lee S, Schonberg MA, Widera E, Smith A. Prognostic indices for older adults: a systematic review. JAMA. 2012;307:182–92.
23. Schonberg MA, Breslau E, McCarthy EP. Targeting of mammography screening according to life expectancy in women age 75 and older. J Am Geriatr Soc. 2013;61:388–95.

# Bone Health in Older Women

**3**

Thomas Hahn, Jensena Carlson,
Adrienne Hampton, and Sarina Schrager

> **Key Points**
> 1. Bone health is particularly important in older women due to increased risk of osteoporosis.
> 2. Osteoporosis is primarily due to effects of aging and decrease in sex steroids.
> 3. Tobacco and alcohol use can increase risk of osteoporosis.
> 4. Osteoporosis often presents with pathologic fractures of the vertebrae, hip, or radius.
> 5. Routine screening for osteoporosis is recommended at age 65 or earlier in someone with a fragility fracture or other risk factors.
> 6. Calcium and vitamin D supplementation are recommended in postmenopausal women.
> 7. Weight-bearing and resistance exercises are key components of bone health.
> 8. Bisphosphonates are effective first-line treatments for osteoporosis.

> **Case**
> The next patient in your clinic is Ester, a 67-year-old woman with history of chronic kidney disease (CKD) stage 3A, hypertension, chronic obstructive pulmonary disease (COPD), and acid reflux, who is coming in for an annual exam after not being seen for several years. She quit smoking cigarettes

10 years ago and takes lisinopril, inhaled fluticasone, and omeprazole. She walks twice per week and recently started a plant-based diet. When you ask if she has any concerns, she says, "My older sister recently fractured her hip, and I am worried that I might have osteoporosis."

## Definitions

*Osteoporosis* is a disease characterized by low bone density and disordered architecture of the bones.

*Osteopenia* refers to bones that are weakened but not as severely as in osteoporosis.

## Epidemiology and Risk Factors and Pathogenesis

### Epidemiology

Osteoporosis is the most common bone disorder seen in postmenopausal women. Osteoporosis is characterized by low bone density and disordered bone architecture and predisposes to fractures. Latest estimates suggest that close to 10 million Americans have osteoporosis and an additional 43 million have osteopenia [1]. Worldwide, it is estimated that one in three women over age 50 will experience an osteoporotic fracture during their lifetime [2].

The 44 million people in the USA with osteoporosis and osteopenia comprise 55% of people over 50 years of age [2].

### Risk Factors and Pathogenesis

The biggest risk factor for osteoporosis is low bone density. Bone density is determined by peak bone density and rate of bone loss. Peak bone mass is based on genetics and nutritional intake and is achieved by the second or third decade of life and starts to slowly decline around age 30 (Fig. 3.1) [3, 4]. Bone formation is balanced with bone remodeling until menopause when the process becomes uncoupled, causing a rapid decline in bone density.

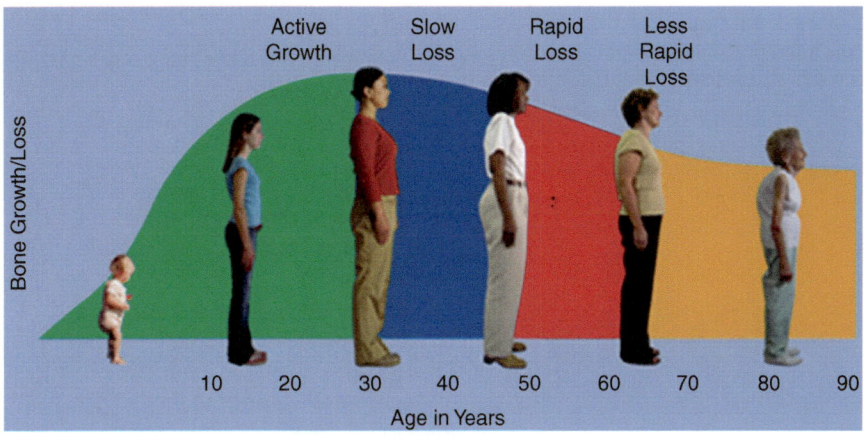

**Fig. 3.1** Bone growth and loss: bone mass starts to decline around age 30, leading to skeletal changes, including kyphosis [5]

**Table 3.1** Fixed risk factors for osteoporosis

| Risk factor |
| --- |
| Age |
| Female gender |
| Family history of osteoporosis or fracture |
| Ethnicity (Caucasian or Asian) |
| Previous fracture |
| Early menopause (<40 years of age) |
| Note: Fixed risk factors for osteoporosis include personal characteristics and fracture history |

> A recent cohort study of almost 6400 people measured bone density tests every 5 years between ages 10 and 25 and found that later age of puberty was correlated with lower peak bone density [6].

Other risk fractures for osteoporosis and fracture can be divided into two groups: fixed risk factors and medical or lifestyle factors (Table 3.1). Osteoporosis is more common in White and Asian women than in African American women.

## Pathophysiology

> Not excited about reading about pathophysiology? Check out this Osmosis video for a helpful 9-minute summary of osteoporosis pathophysiology. https://www.youtube.com/watch?v=jUQ_tt_zJDo&vl=ru [7].

**Table 3.2** Medical conditions that result in secondary osteoporosis [4, 8]

| Medical condition |
| --- |
| Blood disorders (leukemia, multiple myeloma) |
| Chronic kidney disease |
| Chronic obstructive pulmonary disease |
| Cushing's disease |
| Diabetes mellitus |
| Eating disorders (anorexia) |
| Gastrointestinal disorders causing malabsorption (celiac disease) |
| Hyperparathyroidism |
| Hyperthyroidism |
| Liver disease |
| Multiple sclerosis |
| Rheumatoid arthritis |
| Substance use (alcohol and tobacco) |

Note: Multiple medical conditions including pulmonary, endocrine, and gastrointestinal disorders can lead to secondary osteoporosis

Osteoporosis can result from primary and secondary causes. Primary osteoporosis in women is due to bone loss as a result of two things: aging and decrease in sex steroids. During premenopausal years, bone remodeling by osteoblasts creates strong bones, but over time bone resorption from osteoclasts outpaces bone formation by osteoblasts leading to decreased bone formation.

Additionally, aging results in deterioration of the bone microarchitecture and decreased bone mass through bone-intrinsic factors such as oxidative stress, mitochondrial dysfunction, DNA damage, and lipid peroxidation, and also through bone-extrinsic factors such as changes in the immune system and ovaries [3, 4].

Sex hormones including estrogen and androgens help to maintain bone homeostasis by keeping a balance between bone resorption and remodeling. When sex hormones decrease during menopause, this balance becomes off and bone resorption increases [3].

Secondary causes of osteoporosis include medical conditions and use of substances such as tobacco, alcohol, and medications that increase bone resorption and decrease calcium absorption (Tables 3.2 and 3.3).

> **Even Subclinical Hyperthyroidism Increases Fracture Risk** [9]
> A large meta-analysis (total of over 70,000 participants) found that people with subclinical hyperthyroidism (especially among people with a TSH <0.10 mIU/L) were at higher risk of hip and other fractures. This should be considered when assessing overall risk.

# 3 Bone Health in Older Women

**Table 3.3** Medications that increase risk of osteoporosis [10, 11]

| Medication |
|---|
| GnRH agonists |
| Anticonvulsants |
| Tamoxifen (premenopausal) and aromatase inhibitors |
| Chemotherapy drugs |
| Depot medroxyprogesterone acetate (DMPA; bone loss is reversible) |
| Methotrexate |
| Proton pump inhibitors |
| Lithium |
| Antipsychotic medications |

Note: Multiple medications can increase the risk of osteoporosis through decreased calcium absorption and increased bone destruction

### How Glucocorticoids Impact Bone Health
Excess glucocorticoids affect osteoblasts, osteoclasts, and osteocytes by suppressing osteoblastogenesis, which stimulates apoptosis of osteoblasts and osteocytes and increases the lifespan of osteoclasts, leading to increased bone destruction and decreased bone formation [3].

### Case (Continued)
**What Are Ester's Risk Factors for Osteoporosis?**
Age > 65, female, family history of osteoporotic fracture, chronic conditions (CKD, COPD), history of tobacco use, and medications (PPI).

### Case (Continued)
**Clinical Presentation**
When you ask more about why Ester is worried about osteoporosis, she discusses her sister's recent fracture and also mentions that she has been having intermittent knee and shoulder pain over the past year and wonders if this might be due to osteoporosis.

### Myth Buster
Some patient assume they have joint pain caused by osteoporosis and others assume they do not have osteoporosis if they do not have any symptoms. Both are false.

**Table 3.4** Effects of vertebral fractures

| Vertebral fractures can cause |
| --- |
| Chronic pain |
| Kyphosis |
| Increased risk of falls |
| Restrictive lung disease |
| Significant morbidity |
| Decreased quality of life |

Osteoporosis and osteopenia are asymptomatic until a fracture occurs. Fragility or pathologic fractures are the most common presentations of osteoporosis and are fractures that occur spontaneously or as a result of minor trauma such as a fall from standing height that normally would not result in a fracture. The most common pathologic fracture sites are the vertebrae, femoral neck, and distal radius [12, 13].

The most clinically significant fractures are hip fractures, but vertebral fractures can cause chronic pain and disability as well (Table 3.4). Hip fractures are associated with significant excess mortality and disability. Only 40% of people with a hip fracture regain their pre-fracture level of independence and up to 20% will never leave a long-term care facility after a fracture [10].

## Screening and Diagnosis

> **Case (Continued)**
> Ester has never had osteoporosis screening but would like to be screened due to her family history. Does she qualify for screening, and if so, what screening options would you recommend for her?

## Screening

> **Short and Sweet: Who to Screen for Osteoporosis?**
> All women >65 years old and all women >50 years old who sustain a fragility fracture or whose osteoporosis risk using the Fracture Risk Assessment Tool (FRAX) is equal to that of a 65-year-old woman.

Osteoporosis screening with a direct bone density measurement should be considered in all women aged 65 and older regardless of risk factors according to the United States Preventive Services Task Force (USPSTF) [14]. These guidelines are based on evidence that though there is a rapid loss of bone mineral density (BMD) in the lumbar spine in all women after menopause, the risk of fracture does not begin to increase exponentially until age 70–79 [15].

There is less clear evidence regarding screening younger postmenopausal women for osteoporosis, in particular, which risk factors to consider and at what age to begin screening. A 2010 comparison review of screening instruments demonstrated that most include similar considerations and are generally equivalent in predicting fracture risk, regardless of the instrument complexity [16]. The USPSTF suggests using the FRAX to determine a patient's risk for osteoporosis and consider screening women at an earlier age who have a 10-year fracture risk that is equal to a 65-year-old white woman without additional risk factors (8.4% for a woman of mean height and weight) in conjunction with a shared decision-making conversation with the patient [14, 16]. The American Association of Clinical Endocrinologists (AACE)/American College of Endocrinology (ACE) recommends evaluating all premenopausal women age ≥ 50 utilizing a tool such as the FRAX or Osteoporosis Self-assessment Tool (OST) [17].

> *Check out the interactive FRAX at this link*: https://www.sheffield.ac.uk/FRAX/ [18]

What is clear is that all women who sustain a "fragility fracture," a fracture that occurs in the absence of significant trauma, over age 50 should be evaluated with a bone density measurement to evaluate for osteoporosis [11].

## Screening Methods

> **Short and Sweet: How to Screen?**
> Dual energy X-ray absorptiometry (DEXA) scan is the gold standard for screening.

## Screening Methods (Table 3.5)

*DEXA* is the gold standard for bone mineral density (BMD) measurement as it directly measures the bone density at the vertebra and femur. In the DEXA scan, energy from two low-dose X-ray beams passes through and is absorbed by bones, and the energy that is not absorbed is detected on the other side of the body. Bones that are denser absorb more energy so less energy is detected. The amount of radiation exposure is similar to that from a single chest X-ray [19].

> *Watch this video to understand how a DEXA scan works*: https://www.youtube.com/watch?v=7EkK1oMK5A8 [20]

**Table 3.5** Screening methods for osteoporosis

| Method | Pros | Cons |
| --- | --- | --- |
| Dual energy X-ray absorptiometry (DEXA) | Direct measurement of vertebral and femoral bone density<br>Well studied | Radiation exposure<br>Accessibility |
| pDEXA | Direct measurement of bone density<br>Portable | Radiation<br>Not currently correlated with thresholds for treatment |
| Calcaneal ultrasound | Predicts osteoporosis-related fracture<br>Portable<br>Less expensive | Does not directly measure bone density<br>Not currently correlated with thresholds for treatment |

Note: There are multiple ways to screen for osteoporosis. DEXA is the gold standard, though it is not portable

*Peripheral DEXA* (pDEXA) is similar to central DEXA but measures the BMD at peripheral sites. The measurement devices are portable, which may increase access, and limited data have corroborated its efficacy in identifying osteoporosis. However, it has not been correlated with central DEXA to validate treatment thresholds [14].

*Calcaneal ultrasound* predicts osteoporosis-related fracture and is generally more portable and less expensive than DEXA. However, it does not directly measure the BMD, nor does it correlate strongly with DEXA, which is the foundation for medication treatment thresholds that have shown efficacy [14].

Most national guidelines do not include vertebral imaging (plain films) as a standard recommendation for osteoporosis screening. The National Osteoporosis Foundation (NOF) suggests to consider plain films to screen for occult vertebral fractures in certain populations: (1) women over age 70 with normal T-score; (2) women over age 65 with osteopenia; and (3) postmenopausal women over age 50 with risks (fragility fracture, loss of height, or glucocorticoid treatment) [11].

> **What About Labs?**
> Biochemical markers of bone remodeling are not a standard screening recommendation. These markers may be useful in high-risk groups or in monitoring for response to treatment; however, further evidence is needed [21]. Screening for secondary causes of osteoporosis with tests like serum calcium, vitamin D, creatinine, glucose, parathyroid hormone, and thyroid stimulating hormone may be appropriate in postmenopausal women with risk factors such as high-risk medications, strong family history of osteoporosis, and history of fragility fracture.

There are minimal data regarding the harms of osteoporosis screening; these may include radiation exposure, depending on the method, and opportunity cost [14]. There is one study demonstrating that screening does not impact anxiety levels or quality of life [22].

## Diagnosis

Bone density results are reported with a T-score, which indicates bone density relative to the bone density of a healthy 30-year-old woman. Normal bone density is above −1 and low bone density is −1 and below.

> *Osteoporosis*: Fragility fracture *or* T-score < −2.5 at the lumbar spine, femoral neck, or total femur (use the lowest T-score).

> *Osteopenia*: Low normal bone density defined as T-score between −1 and −2.5 at the lumbar spine, femoral neck, or total femur (use the lowest T-score).

> **Case (Continued)**
> Ester elects to have a DEXA scan. Her results show that her lowest T-score is at her femoral neck and is −2.0 and she has a 10-year probability of hip fracture of 1% and 10-year probability of major osteoporotic fracture of 10%. She is diagnosed with osteopenia and asks, "When do I need to have this test repeated?"

> **How Often Should Women Be Screened for Osteoporosis?**
> The optimal frequency of bone density measurement has not been determined, although two large studies demonstrated minimal additional benefit in predicting future fractures with a repeat screening at either 4 or 8 years for women not treated with bisphosphonates [23, 24]. For patients on medication therapy for osteoporosis, the National Osteoporosis Foundation recommends BMD testing 1–2 years after starting treatment and then every 2 years [12].

## Prevention and Management

### Prevention and Lifestyle Treatments

> **Case (Continued)**
> Ester is relieved that she does not have osteoporosis but is worried about her osteopenia and wants to do everything possible to prevent it from progressing to osteoporosis. She would like to avoid taking medication if possible but is eager to lead a healthy lifestyle. What options you would suggest to Ester?

**Table 3.6** Lifestyle preventive treatments for osteoporosis

| Treatment |
|---|
| Well-balanced diet |
| Calcium (1200 mg) and vitamin D (800 IU) supplementation (or diet high in calcium and vitamin D) |
| Weight-bearing and resistance exercises |
| Tai Chi and yoga |
| Fall prevention |

Note: A healthy lifestyle, including nutrition and physical activity, is an important part of maintaining adequate bone health and preventing osteoporosis

Primary prevention of osteoporosis begins with achieving adequate peak bone density in adolescence and early adulthood through optimal nutrition and physical activity. Later in adulthood, primary prevention centers around maintaining bone mass and healthy skeletal microarchitecture. Strategies include adequate nutrition, and weight-bearing and resistance exercises (Table 3.6). Though the data are mixed, the National Osteoporosis Foundation recommends adequate calcium and vitamin D intake in persons over 50 years of age. Standard recommendations for most postmenopausal women with osteoporosis include a total calcium intake of 1000–1500 mg/day and a total vitamin D intake of 600–800 IU per day through diet, supplements, or both [25].

> **When Should You Offer Preventive Medications to Patients with Osteopenia?**
> Preventive medications may be considered in people with osteopenia (T-score between −1.0 and −2.5 at the femoral neck or lumbar spine) and a 10-year probability of a hip fracture ≥3% or a 10-year probability of a major osteoporosis-related fracture ≥20% based on the US adapted WHO algorithm [11].

## Diet

A healthy, well-balanced diet is essential to developing and maintaining healthy bone mineral density and preventing fractures. In postmenopausal women, there is a positive association between higher fruit and vegetable intake and higher bone mineral density with less loss of bone mineral density over time. Fruits and vegetables are important sources of multiple nutrients for bone health, including calcium carotenoids, lycopene, vitamin K, potassium, and magnesium, all of which have demonstrated an inverse relationship with bone turnover, a positive relationship with bone density, or an inverse relationship with fracture risk [26].

> The Framingham osteoporosis study demonstrated that men and women with diets rich in fish (>3 servings per week) over 4 years experienced an increase in bone mineral density, which was not observed in people with only low to moderate fish intake. These findings have been corroborated by multiple cross-sectional cohort studies of bone mineral density in postmenopausal Chinese women as well [26].

Milk and yogurt may have a protective effect against hip fractures, and this effect may be in part mediated by a positive effect of these foods on bone mineral density. Other dairy foods do not appear to affect fracture risk [26].

## Calcium and Vitamin D

The effect of calcium and vitamin D on fracture risk is controversial [26]. Calcium is stored in the bones and adequate calcium stores are essential to healthy bone microarchitecture [27]. Vitamin D3 is necessary for the absorption of calcium from the gut [27]. In a randomized controlled trial of more than 36,000 postmenopausal women, 1000 mg of elemental calcium and 400 international units of vitamin D daily failed to demonstrate a fracture benefit. However, subgroup analysis suggests that women over 60 and women who were adherent to the regimen of calcium and vitamin D did suffer fewer fractures. There are data from populations of institutionalized elderly and elderly people with low dietary calcium and vitamin D intake that corroborate these findings. Therefore, the National Osteoporosis Foundation recommends calcium and vitamin D supplementation in persons over 50 years of age [11]. Standard recommendations for most postmenopausal women with osteoporosis include a total calcium intake of 1000–1500 mg per day, and a total vitamin D intake of 600–800 IU per day through diet, supplements, or both [25].

> **Case (Continued)**
> When you discuss calcium and vitamin D with Ester, she says, "I've heard that calcium can increase my risk of heart disease. Is that true?"

> **Calcium and Cardiovascular Disease**
> There is no evidence to date that *dietary calcium* increases the risk of coronary artery calcification or cardiovascular events. A list of calcium-rich foods can be found here: https://www.iofbonehealth.org/osteoporosis-musculoskeletal-disorders/osteoporosis/prevention/calcium/calcium-content-common-foods [28]
> There is some evidence that if someone is taking *supplemental calcium* and total calcium intake exceeds 1400 mg per day, there may be an increased risk of coronary artery calcification and myocardial infarction [29]. Experts agree that obtaining adequate calcium from food is the preferred way to promote optimal bone and cardiovascular health [29, 30].

## Exercise

Exercise decreases the risk of falls and fractures through improved bone mineral density, improved balance, and decreased risk of falls. The National Osteoporosis Foundation recommends a program of weight-bearing and resistance exercises to prevent falls and fractures, and a sample exercise regimen is available on the NOF website: https://www.nof.org/preventing-fractures/exercise-to-stay-healthy/ [31].

Nonweight-bearing high-force resistance exercises such as strength training for the lower limbs have the most robust evidence for BMD of the femur neck. For BMD of the spine, combined programs comprising more than one exercise type show the most benefit [32].

Tai Chi shows a protective effect against falls, decreasing the risk of falling at least once, and decreasing the rate of falls [33]. Taking part in yoga has been shown to decrease the risk of lower limb fractures [34]. Yoga programs specific to patients with osteoporosis are available.

## Smoking Cessation

First- and second-hand tobacco smoke have a negative effect on bone mass. Tobacco smoke directly affects osteogenesis and bone angiogenesis. Additionally, tobacco smoke mediates indirect effects on bone tissue through alteration of body weight, parathyroid hormone–vitamin D axis, adrenal hormones, sex hormones, and increased oxidative stress. These deleterious effects on skeletal health are largely reversible with tobacco cessation [35].

The Centers for Disease Control and Prevention (CDC) has a smoking cessation website specifically for adults aged 60 and older.

## Alcohol Consumption

The National Osteoporosis Foundation recommends screening for and treating excessive alcohol use (>2 alcoholic beverages per day for women) [11]. Alcohol use in moderation may have a protective effect on bone mineral density. In one study, compared to no consumption, low to moderate alcohol consumption was associated with a lower risk of hip fractures, particularly with red wine consumption among women [36].

## Fall Prevention

Exercise, personalized risk assessment and intervention, and home safety evaluation and modification performed by an occupational therapist all reduce the risk of falls. In people with vitamin D deficiency, vitamin D supplementation may reduce the risk of falls. There is no role for vitamin D supplementation in people with normal vitamin D levels for prevention of falls. Evidence is mixed for the review and management of psychotropic medication for reducing falls. The gradual withdrawal of psychotropic medications may have a positive impact on falls, though evidence for this is most robust when prescribers are supported by drug management protocols [37].

The Centers for Disease Control and Prevention (CDC) has a helpful falls prevention toolkit (Stopping Elderly Accidents, Deaths, and Injuries) for healthcare providers https://www.cdc.gov/steadi/index.html. Many community organizations offer evidence-based falls prevention programs for older adults: the National Council on Aging provides information about how to find these programs in your community https://ncoa.org/ncoa-map.

## Pharmacologic Treatment

**Case (Continued)**
Ester opts to increase calcium in her diet, start calcium and vitamin D supplementation, and introduce Tai Chi and strength training into her weekly routine. She is thankful that she quit smoking 10 years ago. Ester's sister Lucy, who is 70 and recently broke her hip after tripping over a rug in her home, is also your patient and comes to see you for a hospital follow-up visit. She had a normal DEXA scan at age 65 and had not had a repeat scan. You order a DEXA scan, which shows osteoporosis. What treatment would you recommend for Lucy?

**Candidates for Pharmacologic Therapy**
Postmenopausal women and men aged 50 and older presenting with any of the following should be considered for treatment:

1. A hip or vertebral fracture in a patient with osteopenia or osteoporosis.
2. T-score $\leq -2.5$ at the femoral neck, total hip, or lumbar spine.
3. Low bone mass/osteoporosis (T-score between $-1.0$ and $-2.5$ at the femoral neck or lumbar spine) and a 10-year probability of a hip fracture $\geq 3\%$ or a 10-year probability of a major osteoporotic fracture $\geq 20\%$ [18].

Pharmacologic agents for the treatment of osteoporosis have been shown to improve BMD and reduce the risk of fractures. These can be classified as antiresorptive, slowing osteoclast-mediated bone resorption, or anabolic, stimulating osteoblasts to form new bone [11].

## Bisphosphonates

These drugs are FDA approved for the prevention and treatment of osteoporosis, and they are the most prescribed class of drugs for these indications (Table 3.7). They work by inhibiting bone remodeling.

**Table 3.7** Bisphosphonate indications, dosing, and administration

| Drug | Indication | Fracture risk reduction | Dosing | Administration |
|---|---|---|---|---|
| Alendronate | Prevention and treatment of postmenopausal osteoporosis; increase in BMD in men with osteoporosis; treatment of osteoporosis in men and women on glucocorticoid therapy | Reduces the incidence of spine, hip, and vertebral fractures by about 50% over 3 years | Prevention: 5 mg tablet daily or 35 mg tablet weekly<br>Treatment: 10 mg tablet daily; 70 mg tablet weekly; 70 mg tablet weekly with 2800 or 5600 IU of vitamin D3; or 70 mg effervescent tablet weekly | Take with 8 oz of plain water; Binosto® must be dissolved in 4 oz of room temperature water | Oral preparations of these medications must be taken on an empty stomach (except where otherwise noted), first thing in the morning with plain water, no other liquid; after taking these medications, patients must wait at least 30 min before eating, drinking, or taking any other medication; patients should remain upright (sitting or standing) during this time |
| Risedronate | Prevention and treatment of postmenopausal osteoporosis; increase in BMD in men with osteoporosis; treatment of osteoporosis in men and women on glucocorticoid therapy | Reduces the incidence of vertebral fractures by approximately half and nonvertebral fractures by 36% over 3 years; significant risk reduction occurs within 1 year of treatment in patients with a prior vertebral fracture | Prevention and treatment: 5 mg tablet daily; 35 mg tablet weekly; 35 mg delayed release tablet weekly; 35 mg tablet weekly packaged with six tablets of 500 mg calcium carbonate; 75 mg tablets on two consecutive days monthly; and 150 mg tablet monthly | Take with 8 oz of plain water; delayed release risedronate (Atelvia) tablets must be taken immediately after breakfast with at least 4 oz of plain water | |
| Ibandronate | Prevention and treatment of postmenopausal osteoporosis | Reduces the incidence of vertebral fractures by about half over 3 years; no reduction in risk of nonvertebral fractures has not been documented | Prevention: 150 mg tablet monthly<br>Treatment: 150 mg tablet monthly or 3 mg every 3 months by intravenous injection | Take with 8 oz of plain water; serum creatinine should be checked before each injection | |
| Zoledronic acid | Prevention and treatment of postmenopausal osteoporosis; treatment in men with osteoporosis; prevention and treatment of osteoporosis in men and women on glucocorticoid therapy with expected duration ≥12 months | Reduces the incidence of vertebral fractures by 70% (with significant reduction at 1 year), hip fractures by 41%, and nonvertebral fractures by 25% over 3 years | Prevention: 5 mg in 100 mL by intravenous infusion once every 2 years<br>Treatment: 5 mg in 100 mL by intravenous infusion once yearly | Acute phase reaction occurs with approximately one-third of initial injections; risk decreases with subsequent injections; symptoms include arthralgia, headache, myalgia, and fever; patients should be well hydrated and may be pretreated with acetaminophen to reduce the risk of an acute phase reaction | |

Information compiled from Cosman et al. [11]
Note: Bisphosphonates are the first-line medication used to treat osteoporosis. They are effective and overall safe

Use of bisphosphonates should be limited to persons who have an estimated creatinine clearance greater than 35 mL/min. Symptomatic hypocalcemia can develop in patients with low vitamin D levels who are treated with bisphosphonates [25]. Therefore, the National Osteoporosis Foundation recommends screening for and correcting vitamin D deficiency in conjunction with bisphosphonate therapy. The therapeutic target for vitamin D supplementation is 30 ng/mL (75 nmol/L), and maintenance dosing should continue to maintain this level [11].

> **Case (Continued)**
> You and Lucy decide to initiate bisphosphonate therapy for Lucy. When should you start bisphosphonate therapy in a patient with fracture?

> **Initiation of Bisphosphonate Therapy in a Patient After Fracture**
> It is best to wait 4–6 weeks after a fracture before starting bisphosphonate therapy.

Minor gastrointestinal irritation may occur with oral bisphosphonate therapy; this side effect may be minimized by adherence to dosing instructions. It is estimated that less than 40% of persons who are prescribed oral bisphosphonates are still taking them after 1 year. Intravenous preparations with less frequent dosing intervals may therefore be preferred [25].

Rarely, atypical femur fractures and osteonecrosis of the jaw are observed with bisphosphonate therapy. The risk of these complications increases with protracted (>5 years) use. Patients with atypical femur fractures may present with new thigh or groin pain and patients on bisphosphonate therapy should be screened for these symptoms, with bilateral femur X-rays as part of the initial evaluation of these symptoms [11].

> *Medication-related osteonecrosis of the jaw (MRONJ)* is defined as exposed maxillofacial bone for greater than 8 weeks in patients with known exposure to an offending medication and no history of radiation or metastases to the jaw. This primarily occurs in patients on high-dose bisphosphonates for cancer therapy. Denosumab and other antiresorptive agents have also been implicated in the development of MRONJ. Physical examination may reveal exposed bone with no other symptoms. MRONJ requires dental consultation for further evaluation and management [38].

## Estrogen

Estrogen treatment affects osteocytes, osteoclasts, and osteoblasts, causing inhibition of bone resorption and maintenance of bone formation [25]. Estrogen is FDA approved for osteoporosis prevention [11]. In women who have not had a hysterectomy, estrogen is administered with progesterone to prevent endometrial cancer [11]. In the large multicenter Women's Health Initiative trials, estrogen significantly reduced the incidence of new vertebral, nonvertebral, and hip fractures. Estrogen is not recommended as first-line therapy for osteoporosis prevention, in part due to concerns about nonskeletal risks associated with estrogen use including breast cancer and coronary, cerebrovascular, and thrombotic events [25].

## SERMs

Selective estrogen-receptor modulators (SERMs) activate tissue receptors for estrogen that affect bone turnover. Raloxifene is a SERM with FDA approval for the treatment of osteoporosis. It inhibits bone resorption, increases spine BMD, and decreases the risk of vertebral fractures by 30%. Raloxifene has no effect on the risk of hip or other nonvertebral fractures [25]. Like estrogen, Raloxifene increases the risk of deep vein thrombosis. Hot flashes and leg cramps are other commonly observed side effects [11].

## Estrogen/SERM

Conjugated estrogens/bazedoxifene is a combination of estrogen and a SERM approved by the FDA to prevent osteoporosis after menopause. This drug significantly increases mean lumbar spine BMD after a year of therapy as compared to placebo in women who have been postmenopausal between 1 and 5 years. This drug also significantly increases total hip BMD [11].

## Denosumab

Denosumab is a human monoclonal antibody that inhibits bone resorption by inhibiting osteoclasts [25]. Denosumab is approved by the FDA for the treatment of osteoporosis in postmenopausal women at high risk of fracture [11]. This drug lowers risk of vertebral fractures by 68%, hip fractures by 40%, and other nonvertebral fractures by 20% as compared to placebo. It can be used in women with compromised renal function. As with bisphosphonates, rare cases of atypical femur fractures and osteonecrosis of the jaw have been observed with denosumab treatment [25].

## Calcitonin

Calcitonin nasal spray is FDA approved for women who are at least 5 years postmenopausal when other osteoporosis treatments are not appropriate. Calcitonin reduces vertebral fracture occurrence by about 30% in those with prior vertebral fractures but has not been shown to reduce the risk of nonvertebral fractures. Calcitonin may cause rhinitis, epistaxis, and allergic reactions, particularly in those with a history of allergy to salmon. Calcitonin may be associated with malignancy, and need for this therapy should be frequently reassessed [11].

## Teriparatide

Teriparatide (recombinant human parathyroid hormone [$rhPTH$]) stimulates osteoblastic bone formation to increase bone mass and improve bone architecture [39].

Teriparatide is FDA approved for the treatment of osteoporosis in men and postmenopausal women with high risk of fracture, including those with a history of glucocorticoid use [40]. Teriparatide is administered daily by self-injection for 24 months [39]. This drug lowered the risk of vertebral fractures by 65% and non-vertebral fractures by 53% in a large randomized placebo-controlled trial [41]. These benefits persisted beyond the treatment interval. In clinical trials, rare cases of osteosarcoma were observed, though no causal link has been established [39].

## Duration of Therapy

The recommended duration of therapy for bisphosphonates is 3–5 years, after which time a 3–5 year drug holiday is recommended because the potential for additional therapeutic effect wanes and the risk of osteonecrosis of the jaw and atypical femur fractures increases. The benefits of bisphosphonate therapy persist for a few years after discontinuation of therapy. The effects of nonbisphosphonate therapies attenuate rapidly after therapy discontinuation, with the exception of teriparatide [11].

> **Case (Continued)**
> Lucy takes alendronate for 5 years, with improvements seen on interval DEXA scans. Five years after finishing treatment, at age 80, she has a repeat bone density scan, which shows worsening of her osteoporosis. Should she restart the medication?

There is not clear evidence or guidelines about when to restart bisphosphonates after a drug holiday. Patients with risk factors such as decrease in BMD, new fracture, or other clinical risk factors for fracture who were previously treated may benefit from restarting therapy if there has been persistent bone loss (about 5%) on at least two DEXA scans taken at least 2 years apart. Additionally, if a patient with osteoporosis was treated and had a 3–5 year holiday with documented improvement from therapy and no history of fractures, you can also consider restarting therapy [42].

Bone health can have a significant impact on the lives of older women. Healthy bones can pave the way for a healthy, active lifestyle whereas osteoporosis can lead to significant morbidity. Thus, routine bone health risk assessment and screening and discussion of preventive and therapeutic treatment options are very important in order to maximize bone health and quality of life.

## References

1. Wright NC, Looker A, Saag KG, Curtis JR, Dalzell ES, Randal S, Dawson-Hughes B. The recent prevalence of osteoporosis and low bone mass based on bone mineral density at the femoral neck or lumbar spine in the United States. J Bone Min Res. 2014;29(11):2520–6.
2. International osteoporosis foundation, osteoporosis statistics. Available at: https://www.iof-bonehealth.org/facts/statistics#category-23. Accessed 31 Oct 19.

3. Manolagas S. Pathogenesis of osteoporosis. UpToDate. 2019. Updated 03/06/2018. https://www.uptodate.com/contents/pathogenesis-of-osteoporosis?search=osteoporosis%20pathogenesis&source=search_result&selectedTitle=1~150&usage_type=default&display_rank=1. Accessed 01 Nov 2019.
4. Rosen CJ. The epidemiology and pathogenesis of osteoporosis. Endotext. 2017. www.endotext.org. Updated 02/21/2017. Accessed 01 Nov 2019.
5. The surgeon general's report on bone health and osteoporosis: what it means to you. National Institutes of Health Osteoporosis and Related Bone Diseases National Resources Center. (2/2017). Available at, https://www.bones.nih.gov/health-info/bone/SGR/surgeon-generals-report. Accessed 13 Apr 2020.
6. Elhakcem A, Frysz M, Tilling K, Tobias JH, Lawlor DA. Association between age at puberty and bone accrual from 10 to 25 years of age. JAMA Netw Open. 2019;2(8):e198918.
7. Osmosis. Osteoporosis: causes, symptoms, diagnosis, treatment, pathology. July 12, 2019. https://www.youtube.com/watch?v=jUQ_tt_zJDo&vl=ru. . Accessed 13 Apr 2020
8. International Osteoporosis Foundation. Secondary osteoporosis. 2017. https://www.iofbonehealth.org/secondary-osteoporosis. Accessed 24 Nov 2019.
9. Blum RR, Bauer DC, Collet TH, Fink HA, Cappola AR, da Costa BR, et al. Subclinical thyroid dysfunction and fracture risk: a meta-analysis. JAMA. 2015;313(20):2055–65.
10. Office of the Surgeon General (US) Bone health and osteoporosis: a report of the Surgeon General. 2004. Office of the Surgeon General. Available at: http://www.ncbi.nlm.nih.gov/books/NBD45513. Accessed 31 Oct 2019.
11. Cosman F, de Beur SJ, LeBoff MS, Lewiecki EM, Tanner B, Randall S, Lindsay R, (for an expert committee for the National Osteoporosis Foundation). Clinicians guide to prevention and treatment of osteoporosis. Osteoporos Int 2014;25:2359–2381.
12. DynaMed [Internet]. Ipswich: EBSCO Information Services. 1995. Record No. T113815, Osteoporosis; [updated 2018 Dec 03, cited 11/19/2019]. Available from https://www.dynamed.com/topics/dmp~AN~T113815. Registration and login required.
13. Rosen HN, Drezner MD. Clinical manifestations, diagnosis, and evaluation of osteoporosis in postmenopausal women. UpToDate. 2019. Updated 07/11/2019. https://www.uptodate.com/contents/clinical-manifestations-diagnosis-and-evaluation-of-osteoporosis-in-postmenopausal-women?search=osteoporosis&source=search_result&selectedTitle=2~150&usage_type=default&display_rank=2. Accessed 01 Nov 2019.
14. United States Preventive Services Task Force. Screening for osteoporosis to prevent fractures. JAMA. 2018;319(24):2521–31.
15. Ensrud KE, Crandall CJ. Osteoporosis. Ann Intern Med. 2017;167(3):17–32.
16. Nelson HD, et al. Screening for osteoporosis: an update for the U.S. Preventive Services Task Force. Ann Intern Med. 2010;153(2):99–111.
17. Camacho PM, et al. American Association of Clinical Endocrinologists and American College of endocrinology clinical practice guidelines for the diagnosis and treatment of postmenopausal osteoporosis. Endocr Pract. 2016;22(Suppl 4):1–42.
18. Centre for Metabolic Bone Diseases, University of Sheffield, UK. Fracture risk assessment tool. 2008. https://www.sheffield.ac.uk/FRAX/. Accessed 13 Apr 2020.
19. Berger A. Bone mineral density scans. BMJ. 2002;31(325):7362.
20. Medflox.com. DEXA-Dual Energy X-ray Absorptiometry. July 21, 2008. https://www.youtube.com/watch?v=7EkK1oMK5A8. Accessed 13 Apr 2020.
21. Burch J, et al. Systematic review of the use of bone turnover markers treatment: the secondary prevention of fractures, and primary prevention of fractures in high-risk groups. Health Technol Assess. 2014;18(11):1–180.
22. Shepstone L, et al. Screening in the community to reduce fractures in older women (SCOOP): a randomised controlled trial. Lancet. 2018;391(10122):741–7.
23. Hiller TA, et al. Evaluating the Value of repeat bone mineral density measurement and prediction of fractures in older women. Arch Intern Med. 2007;167:155–60.
24. Berry SD, et al. Repeat bone mineral density screening and prediction of hip and major osteoporotic fracture. JAMA. 2013;310(12):1256–62.

25. Black DM, Rosen CJ. Clinical practice. Postmenopausal osteoporosis. N Engl J Med. 2016;374(3):254–62. https://doi.org/10.1056/NEJMcp1513724.
26. Sahni S, Mangano KM, McLean RR, Hannan MT, Kiel DP. Dietary approaches for bone health: lessons from the Framingham Osteoporosis Study. Curr Osteoporos Rep. 2015;13(4):245–55. https://doi.org/10.1007/s11914-015-0272-1.
27. Vannucci L, Fossi C, Quattrini S, et al. Calcium intake in bone health: a focus on calcium-rich mineral waters. Nutrients. 2018;10(12):1930. https://doi.org/10.3390/nu10121930. Published 2018 Dec 5.
28. https://www.iofbonehealth.org/osteoporosis-musculoskeletal-disorders/osteoporosis/prevention/calcium/calcium-content-common-foods
29. Anderson JJ, Kruszka B, Delaney JA, et al. Calcium intake from diet and supplements and the risk of coronary artery calcification and its progression among older adults: 10-year follow-up of the Multi-Ethnic Study of Atherosclerosis (MESA). J Am Heart Assoc. 2016;5(10):e003815. https://doi.org/10.1161/JAHA.116.003815. Published 2016 Oct 11.
30. National Osteoporosis Foundation. NOF response to report in the Journal of the American Heart Association that calcium supplements may damage the heart. 2016. Osteoporosis in the News. https://www.nof.org/news/nof-response-report-journal-american-heart-association-calcium-supplements-may-damage-heart/. Accessed 3 Dec 2019.
31. https://www.nof.org/preventing-fractures/exercise-to-stay-healthy/
32. Howe TE, Shea B, Dawson LJ, Downie F, Murray A, Ross C, Harbour RT, Caldwell LM, Creed G. Exercise for preventing and treating osteoporosis in postmenopausal women. Cochrane Database Syst Rev. 2011;7:CD000333. https://doi.org/10.1002/14651858.CD000333.pub2.
33. Huang ZG, Feng YH, Li YH, Lv CS. Systematic review and meta-analysis: Tai Chi for preventing falls in older adults. BMJ Open. 2017;7(2):e013661. https://doi.org/10.1136/bmjopen-2016-013661. Published 2017 Feb 6.
34. Armstrong ME, Lacombe J, Wotton CJ, Cairns BJ, Green J, Floud S, Beral V, Reeves GK. The associations between seven different types of physical activity and the incidence of fracture at seven sites in healthy postmenopausal UK women. J Bone Miner Res. 2019. Accepted Author Manuscript. https://doi.org/10.1002/jbmr.3896.
35. Al-Bashaireh AM, Haddad LG, Weaver M, Chengguo X, Kelly DL, Yoon S. The effect of tobacco smoking on bone mass: an overview of pathophysiologic mechanisms. J Osteoporos. 2018;2018, 17 pp. https://doi.org/10.1155/2018/1206235.
36. Fung TT, Mukamal KJ, Rimm EB, Meyer HE, Willett WC, Feskanich D. Alcohol intake, specific alcoholic beverages, and risk of hip fractures in postmenopausal women and men age 50 and older. Am J Clin Nutr. 2019;110(3):691–700. https://doi.org/10.1093/ajcn/nqz135.
37. Gillespie LD, Robertson MC, Gillespie WJ, Sherrington C, Gates S, Clemson LM, Lamb SE. Interventions for preventing falls in older people living in the community. Cochrane Database Syst Rev. 2012;9:CD007146. https://doi.org/10.1002/14651858.CD007146.pub3.
38. Ruggiero SL, Dodson TB, Fantasia J, et al. American Association of Oral and Maxillofacial Surgeons position paper on medication-related osteonecrosis of the jaw–2014 update. J Oral Maxillofac Surg. 2014;72:1938–56.
39. Lindsay R, Krege JH, Marin F, Jin L, Stepan JJ. Teriparatide for osteoporosis: importance of the full course. Osteoporos Int. 2016;27(8):2395–410. https://doi.org/10.1007/s00198-016-3534-6.
40. US Food and Drug Administration Website. https://www.accessdata.fda.gov/drugsatfda_docs/nda/2002/21-318_FORTEO_Approv.pdf. Accessed 3 Dec 2019.
41. Neer RM, Arnaud CD, Zanchetta JR, Prince R, Gaich GA, Reginster JY, Hodsman AB, Eriksen EF, Ish-Shalom S, Genant HK, Wang O, Mitlak BH. Effect of parathyroid hormone (1–34) on fractures and bone mineral density in postmenopausal women with osteoporosis. N Engl J Med. 2001;344(19):1434–41.
42. Rosen HN. The use of bisphosphonates in postmenopausal women with osteoporosis. UpToDate. UpToDate.com. Updated 07/10/2019. Accessed 15 Nov 2019.

# Depression and Grief in Older Women

## 4

Julia Lubsen, Jillian Landeck, and Melissa Stiles

**Key Points**
- Depression in older adults can present with mainly physical symptoms and/or behavioral changes.
- Evaluate for medical causes of symptoms of depression and cognitive impairment.
- Nonpharmacologic treatments like psychotherapy are beneficial in the treatment of older women with depression and grief and are often preferred.
- There are specific antidepressants that are safer in older women.
- When prescribing antidepressants, "start low, go slow, and keep going" until therapeutic effect is achieved. Monitor carefully for side effects.
- Distinguish between normal and complicated grief, and offer psychotherapy and pharmacotherapy as indicated.

**Case 1**
Avis is an 87-year-old woman who is brought to your clinic by her daughter because she has been sleeping most of the day and does not seem like herself. She has given up quilting and no longer wants to meet her friends for Sunday brunch.

You are concerned that she may have depression, but also want to rule out other causes of her symptoms.

---

J. Lubsen (✉) · J. Landeck · M. Stiles
Department of Family Medicine and Community Health, University of Wisconsin School of Medicine and Public Health, Madison, WI, USA
e-mail: julia.lubsen@fammed.wisc.edu; jillian.landeck@fammed.wisc.edu; melissa.stiles@fammed.wisc.edu

**How common is depression in older women like Avis?**
- Clinically significant depressive symptoms are common in later life and affect 10–15% of people aged 55 and older. Minor depression affects 10% of older adults and major depression affects 2% [1, 2].
- The lifetime prevalence of depression is almost two times higher in women than men [3].
- Some groups of older adults have much higher rates of depression. The prevalence of depression is 25% in elders with chronic medical illness and 25–50% in nursing home residents [4].
- The risk of suicide attempts is higher in women, but the risk of suicide completion is lower in women [5].
- Depression is not a part of normal aging. The diagnosis and treatment of depression is important to decrease suffering and improve function and quality of life in older women. Up to 80% of patients achieve remission with appropriate treatment [4].

**What questions would you ask Avis to assess her symptoms?**
- The diagnostic criteria for depression are the same in older and younger people (Box 4.1). You should ask about the typical symptoms of depression, including depressed mood and anhedonia. Here is a quick reference: MD-Calc: DSM-5 Criteria for Major Depressive Disorder.
- Some women may not meet the diagnostic criteria for depression, but still have significant depressive symptoms. Minor depression is usually defined as the presence of one of the two major symptoms of depression (depressed mood, anhedonia) plus one to three additional symptoms. Dysthymia (persistent depressive disorder) is also less severe than major depression and lasts for 2 or more years [4].
- Older women with depression may not report depressed mood. Patients often present with physical symptoms or changes in behavior. In addition to asking about sleep, appetite, and energy level, you should ask about pain, memory problems, and other unexplained physical symptoms. Check for weight loss or weight gain.

**Box 4.1 DSM-5 Diagnostic Criteria for Major Depressive Episode**

Five (or more) of the following symptoms have been present during the same 2-week period:

- Depressed mood (e.g., feels sad, empty, hopeless; appears tearful)
- Markedly diminished interest or pleasure in all, or almost all, activities
- Significant weight loss/gain or change in appetite
- Insomnia or hypersomnia
- Psychomotor agitation or retardation
- Fatigue or loss of energy
- Feelings of worthlessness or excessive or inappropriate guilt
- Diminished ability to think or concentrate, or indecisiveness
- Recurrent thoughts of death, suicidal ideation, or a suicide attempt or a specific plan for committing suicide

At least one of the symptoms is either (1) depressed mood or (2) loss of interest or pleasure.

Symptoms represent a change from previous functioning and cause clinically significant distress or impairment in social, occupational, or other important areas of functioning.

There has never been a manic episode or a hypomanic episode.

Note: Do not include symptoms that are clearly attributable to another medical condition,* the physiological effects of a substance, or another psychiatric disorder such as schizoaffective disorder, schizophrenia, schizophreniform disorder, delusional disorder, or other psychotic disorders.

Adapted from the *Diagnostic and Statistical Manual of Mental Disorders, Fifth Edition* (DSM-5).

*Since depression commonly manifests with physical symptoms in older adults, many geriatric psychiatrists suggest that symptoms should be counted toward the diagnosis regardless of other possible medical explanations [4].

- Take a careful social history.
  - Ask about recent life events, losses, and stressors.
  - Depression can present with significant functional impairment in older adults. Ask about activities of daily living and functional status. Try using the Katz Index of Independence in Activities of Daily Living (ADL) and the Lawton Instrumental Activities of Daily Living (IADL) Scale.
  - Ask about the patient's living environment and social support system.
  - Ask about alcohol and other substance use.
- Explore whether the patient is withdrawing from social activities, refusing to eat or drink, refusing medications, or having difficulty caring for themselves. It can be helpful to get collateral information from a family member or caregiver.
- Assess the patient for delusions and hallucinations, which can be signs of delusional or psychotic depression that requires specialized treatment.
- Consider screening for elder abuse. The Elder Abuse Suspicion Index is one tool that may be used for screening.

| Elder Abuse Suspicion Index (EASI) | |
| --- | --- |
| Questions 1–5 answered by patient; Question 6 answered by doctor *Within the last 12 months*: | |
| 1. Have you relied on people for any of the following: bathing, dressing, shopping, banking, or meals? | Yes No Did not answer |
| 2. Has anyone prevented you from getting food, clothes, medication, glasses, hearing aids, or medical care, or from being with people you wanted to be with? | Yes No Did not answer |
| 3. Have you been upset because someone talked to you in a way that made you feel shamed or threatened? | Yes No Did not answer |
| 4. Has anyone tried to force you to sign papers or to use your money against your will? | Yes No Did not answer |
| 5. Has anyone made you afraid, touched you in ways that you did not want, or hurt you physically? | Yes No Did not answer |
| 6. Doctor: Elder abuse may be associated with findings such as: poor eye contact, withdrawn nature, malnourishment, hygiene issues, cuts, bruises, inappropriate clothing, or medication compliance issues. Did you notice any of these today or in the last 12 months? | Yes No Did not answer |
| The EASI was developed to raise a doctor's suspicion about elder abuse to a level at which it might be reasonable to propose a referral for further evaluation by social services, adult protective services, or equivalents. While all six questions should be asked, a response of "yes" on one or more of questions 2–6 may establish concern. | |

- Ask about the person's past history of psychiatric disorders (depression, bipolar disorder, manic episodes, anxiety, psychosis) and psychiatric hospitalizations. Also ask about family history of psychiatric disorders.

## Assessment Tips

- *Depression in older adults can present with mainly physical symptoms.*
- *Interview the patient's caregiver, especially for older adults with cognitive impairment.*
- *Obtain a detailed social history.*

> **Case 1 (Continued)**
> Avis has lost 10 lbs. in the past 6 months. She tells you that she has difficulty sleeping due to chronic shoulder pain. You discover that she recently lost a close friend. Avis was in the hospital 3 months ago for a fall and pneumonia and had to go to a nursing home for rehab. She still needs to use a walker and has not been able to leave her house without help. Her children have been helping her with shopping and housekeeping. She has never been diagnosed with a psychiatric disorder, but her father struggled with depression.

Avis has several risk factors that increase her risk for depression. Table 4.1 gives examples of risk factors and triggers for depression in older women.

**What tools can you use to assess Avis's depression symptoms?**
- Perform a mental status examination.
- You can use the Patient Health Questionnaire-9 (PHQ-9) or the Geriatric Depression Scale (GDS) to assess depression symptoms and track symptoms over time.

**Table 4.1** Risk factors and triggers for depression in older women

| | |
|---|---|
| Demographics | Age > 85, female sex, family history of depression [2] |
| Psychological | Cognitive impairment, personality disorders, personal history of depression |
| Social | Stressful life events, retirement, financial difficulty, grief, trauma, functional impairment, loss of independence, social isolation, nursing home placement, awareness of mortality |
| Medical conditions | Chronic illness (stroke, cancer, diabetes, heart disease, lung disease), sexual dysfunction, incontinence, falls, frailty, hospitalization |
| Medications/ substances | Chemotherapy, corticosteroids, antiparkinsonian medications, metoclopramide, interferon, various cardiovascular and antihypertensive medications, alcohol [4] |

- Since depression and anxiety commonly occur together, you can use the General Anxiety Disorder-7 (GAD-7) scale to assess anxiety symptoms.

- It is very important to conduct a suicide risk assessment. MD-Calc: Columbia Suicide Severity Rating Scale. Consider psychiatric hospitalization if patient is at high risk for suicide.

### Case 1 (Continued)
Avis has a score of 13 on the PHQ-9 and 11 on the GAD-7, suggesting moderate depression and anxiety. She has been struggling to take care of herself at home. This could be from physical limitations and depression, but you want to make sure that she is not developing cognitive impairment.

**How can you distinguish depression from dementia?**

You assess Avis's cognition using the Mini-Cog. She remembers two out of three words and draws a normal clock (score = 4, normal screen).

Cognitive evaluation is an important part of evaluating depressive symptoms in older adults.
- Older adults with depression can have varying degrees of cognitive impairment, which sometimes improves when depression is treated. Depression is associated with an increased risk of developing dementia later in life. Depression can also develop in people with dementia [4].
- There are several brief cognitive screens available. The Mini-Cog includes a three-item recall (3 points) and clock-draw test (2 points). This can be administered in less than 5 min. A score of 3 or less is abnormal and requires further testing.
- If the Mini-Cog is abnormal, you should perform a more detailed cognitive evaluation such as the Mini-Mental State Examination (MMSE: proprietary), the St. Louis University Mental Status Examination (SLUMS) or the Montreal Cognitive Assessment (MOCA).

### Case 1 (Continued)
Avis has reported fatigue, difficulty sleeping, pain, and weight loss. You wonder if some of her symptoms could be explained by a medical problem. How do you distinguish depression from other medical problems?

- Look for other medical causes of the patient's symptoms (Table 4.2). For example, Avis's fatigue could be caused by sleep apnea, another sleep disorder, sedating medications, hypothyroidism, heart failure, or another medical problem.
- You should carefully review her medication list for medications that could be contributing to her symptoms. Ask about over-the-counter medications including sleep aids, decongestants, antihistamines, and NSAIDs.
- Perform a physical exam relevant to her symptoms.
- Consider checking labs, for example a complete blood count (CBC) to evaluate for anemia, thyroid stimulating hormone (TSH) level to evaluate for thyroid disease, and basic metabolic panel to assess for renal impairment, hyponatremia, and diabetes.
- A basic metabolic panel (BMP) can also be helpful because some antidepressants require dose adjustments or are contraindicated in renal impairment, and many antidepressants can cause hyponatremia during treatment, especially in the elderly.
- Neuroimaging may be useful if the patient has an abnormal neurologic examination suggesting cerebrovascular disease or significant cognitive impairment.

MRI is usually preferred because it is more sensitive than CT for a broad range of pathologies.

> **Case 1 (Continued)**
> Avis's physical exam is normal. She recently had a normal CBC, BMP, and TSH in the hospital. Her daughter says she does snore sometimes, so you order a sleep study to rule out sleep apnea as the cause of her symptoms. You discover that she takes Tylenol PM (acetaminophen with diphenhydramine) for shoulder pain at night. You discuss that the diphenhydramine could be contributing to her fatigue and ask her to switch to plain acetaminophen and topical lidocaine for pain.

> **Case 1 (Continued)**
> You see Avis back in 1 week. Her sleep study was normal. Her pain is well controlled. You discuss treatment options for depression. She would rather not start a medication. What nonpharmacologic treatment options for depression would you discuss with Avis?

**Table 4.2** Differential diagnosis for symptoms of depression

| Symptom | Differential diagnosis | Examples of contributing medications |
|---|---|---|
| Weight loss, decreased appetite | Decreased taste/smell<br>Dental problems<br>Dysphagia<br>Gastritis/peptic ulcer disease<br>Celiac disease<br>Inflammatory bowel disease<br>Microscopic colitis<br>Advanced cardiac/pulmonary disease<br>Adrenal insufficiency<br>Cancer<br>Diabetes<br>Hyperthyroidism<br>Infectious diseases<br>Eating disorder/dietary restrictions<br>Alcohol use disorder<br>Elder abuse/neglect | Antibiotics<br>Anticonvulsants<br>Antidepressants (bupropion, SSRIs)<br>Digoxin<br>Donepezil<br>Metformin<br>Stimulants<br>Thyroid medication (overtreatment)<br>NSAIDs<br>Opioids |
| Insomnia | Alcohol use<br>Caffeine use<br>Nicotine use<br>Gastroesophageal reflux disease<br>Nocturia<br>Menopause<br>Restless leg syndrome<br>Pain<br>Pruritus<br>Hyperthyroidism<br>Sleep apnea | Bronchodilators<br>Antidepressants (bupropion, fluoxetine)<br>Diuretics<br>Glucocorticoids<br>Stimulants<br>Thyroid medication (overtreatment) |
| Fatigue | Advanced cardiac/pulmonary disease<br>Adrenal insufficiency<br>Anemia<br>Hypothyroidism<br>Infectious disease<br>Sleep apnea<br>Renal failure | Anticholinergics<br>Antihistamines<br>Antidepressants (paroxetine)<br>Benzodiazepines<br>Beta-blockers<br>Gabapentin<br>Opioids<br>Sedative hypnotics |

*Source*: Gaddey [6]

- Psychotherapy can be recommended as first-line treatment for mild to moderate depression in the elderly. Psychotherapy can also be combined with medication for moderate to severe depression. There are many types of psychotherapy; cognitive behavioral therapy is the most studied and is effective.
- Exercise therapy can be beneficial if patients can safely exercise.
- Light therapy can be considered, especially for seasonal affective disorder.

> **Case 1 (Continued)**
> Avis starts seeing a counselor and tries to walk around her house for 10 min per day. One month later, Avis is not feeling much better and is interested in discussing medication.

Older adults often need the same doses of antidepressants as younger adult patients, but they are frequently given doses that are subtherapeutic. When prescribing antidepressants to older patients, remember the mantra *"start low, go slow, but keep going"* until a therapeutic effect is achieved.

## What factors should you keep in mind when choosing antidepressants for older women?

- Antidepressant medication should be considered in older patients with moderate to severe depression (PHQ > 10).
- The response rate to antidepressants is almost 50% in patients 55 and older, but their efficacy decreases with increasing age.
- The elderly are at higher risk for adverse events from medications due to comorbid medical conditions and drug–drug interactions. Monitor carefully for side effects.
- Polypharmacy (taking multiple medications) is common in the elderly and can increase the risk of side effects and drug interactions from antidepressants, especially in frail patients. The 2019 Beers Criteria [8] and the 2015 STOPP/START Criteria [9] identify potentially inappropriate medications for older adults. Deprescribing, or discontinuing nonessential medications, can reduce the risks of polypharmacy.
- The older antidepressant classes, tricyclic antidepressants (TCAs) and monoamine oxidase inhibitors (MAOIs), are rarely used due to side effects and safety concerns.
- *Selective serotonin reuptake inhibitors (SSRIs)* are often prescribed first-line because of their relative safety and efficacy. Among the SSRIs, *sertraline, escitalopram*, and *citalopram* are preferred in the elderly because they have fewer side effects and drug interactions. Use *fluoxetine* with caution as it can be overstimulating and has many drug interactions. *Paroxetine* should be avoided in the elderly as it is highly sedating and causes anticholinergic side effects (dry mouth, constipation, urinary retention, confusion).
- *Serotonin norepinephrine reuptake inhibitors (SNRIs)* and other antidepressants (*bupropion* and *mirtazapine*) can also be prescribed. SNRIs can be beneficial for pain. Mirtazapine may be beneficial in older adults who have insomnia and decreased appetite.
- Many antidepressants require dose adjustments based on renal function, or are contraindicated in renal failure; renal function should be monitored. Most antidepressants can cause hyponatremia, especially in the elderly; periodically monitor sodium as well. (Table 4.3)

**Table 4.3** Medications for depression in the elderly

| Category | Major side effects | Medications | Special considerations |
|---|---|---|---|
| **Selective serotonin reuptake inhibitors (SSRIs)**  *First line* | Headache<br>GI upset<br>GI bleeding<br>Weight loss<br>Insomnia<br>Sedation<br>Sexual dysfunction<br>Hyponatremia<br>Prolonged QT<br>Falls<br>Serotonin syndrome | Sertraline | |
| | | Escitalopram | |
| | | Citalopram | Check QTc for doses > 20 mg |
| | | Fluoxetine | Use with caution due to drug-drug interactions, long half-life |
| | | Paroxetine | Avoid in the elderly. Highly anticholinergic and sedating |
| **Serotonin norepinephrine reuptake inhibitors (SNRIs)** | Similar to SSRIs<br>Can increase blood pressure | Venlafaxine | Short half-life, taper slowly to avoid withdrawal, difficult to discontinue |
| | | Duloxetine | May improve pain |
| **Dopamine/norepinephrine reuptake inhibitor** | Headache<br>GI upset<br>Insomnia<br>Weight loss<br>Hyponatremia | Bupropion | Causes less sexual dysfunction than SSRIs/SNRIs |
| **Alpha-2 antagonist** | Sedation<br>Weight gain<br>Hyponatremia | Mirtazapine | Increases appetite and sleep |

Lexicomp, 2019 Beers Criteria [7, 8]
Green = okay to use in the elderly, Yellow = use with caution, Red = avoid use in the elderly

- Antidepressants can take 4–6 weeks to have a therapeutic effect, and it may take much longer to reach a therapeutic dose. Only 1/3 of older adults treated with an antidepressant achieve remission. [2]
- If initial medical therapy does not work, you have the following options:
  - Incorporate nonpharmacologic treatments.
  - Titrate to the maximum adult dose of the initial medication.
  - Switch to a different medication in the same class or a medication from a different class.
  - Add a second antidepressant from a different class.
  - Augment with lithium or atypical antipsychotics (in consultation with psychiatry).
- Patients who have failed two adequate trials of medication therapy have treatment-resistant depression.
- *Electroconvulsive therapy (ECT)* can be a very effective treatment for depression in the elderly. Response rates are much higher with ECT (80–90%) and symptoms improve more quickly compared to medication therapy [2].
  - Indications for ECT include the following:

    Severe or treatment-resistant depression
    Psychotic depression
    Catatonic depression
    Severe malnutrition or a medical condition that worsens because the patient refuses to take medication

  - ECT is relatively safe, but does require general anesthesia and can cause short-term cognitive impairment.
- *Transcranial Magnetic Stimulation (TMS)* has not been well studied in the geriatric population.
- Consider referring to psychiatry for complicated cases including treatment-resistant depression, difficulty tolerating medications, high suicide risk, bipolar disorder, psychosis, and diagnostic uncertainty.

**Case 1 (Continued)**
Avis is prescribed sertraline 25 mg once daily. At her monthly follow-up visits she is improving, but still symptomatic, so sertraline is gradually increased to 100 mg daily. Six months later, Avis returns again and is doing much better. She asks if she can stop her medication.

**Case 2**
Avis's sister, Betty, comes to see you later that year for a diabetes follow-up visit. She usually comes in with her blood sugar log, but today she is embarrassed that she has not been checking her sugars. As you ask her more about that she breaks down in tears and tells you that her husband passed away last month. How would you respond?

**Table 4.4** Timing of discontinuation of antidepressants

| Episodes of depression | When to consider discontinuing antidepressants |
|---|---|
| One | After 1 year in remission |
| Two | After 2 years in remission |
| Three or more | After 3 years in remission, or continue indefinitely |

### When would you advise discontinuing antidepressant medication?
- For a single episode of depression antidepressant medication should be continued for at least 1 year after remission is achieved, based on expert opinion. (Table 4.4) [2]
- In addition to expert guidelines, you should consider patient preference, severity of episodes, difficulty of achieving remission, and risk factors for recurrence when deciding whether to discontinue medications.
- Gradually taper medications and monitor the patient carefully for recurrence of symptoms. Medications should be tapered over at least 4 weeks, and many patients will need a much longer taper to avoid a withdrawal syndrome. Symptoms of withdrawal can include mood changes, flu-like symptoms, insomnia, hyperarousal, nausea, balance impairment, and sensory disturbances. Paroxetine and venlafaxine have short half-lives, contributing to significant withdrawal symptoms if they are stopped abruptly.

### How to talk to someone experiencing grief:
- All clinicians have an opportunity to provide compassionate care to patients experiencing grief and direct them to additional resources.
- Discussions with grieving individuals should be warm, inviting, and open ended. It is important to try to be present without trying to fix the problem.
- It can be helpful to preface difficult conversations about loss with a statement such as, "Although I speak with a lot of people who have experienced the loss of a loved one, each person's experience is unique. I would like to talk to you more about what you are going through."
- Try to begin this difficult conversation by asking about the person who died, the specific circumstances around their death, and how they have been coping since their death (e.g., how the loss is affecting their emotions, daily activities, social interactions, and work).
- It is then important to ask about their support system and the effectiveness of this support system.

### How are bereavement and grief defined?
Bereavement is the experience of losing a loved one to death. Grief is the response to bereavement, which comprises a variety of emotional and physical symptoms and

signs that fluctuate over time and vary greatly between individuals [10]. Culture, ethnicity, gender and spiritual beliefs greatly influence one's experience and strategies for coping with grief.

> Typical symptoms of acute grief include the following:
> - Intense yearning, longing, sorrow, emotional pain, physical symptoms, abdominal discomfort, frequent yawning, dizziness/fogginess
> - Feelings of disbelief, difficulty comprehending the reality of the death
> - Insistent distracting thoughts of the deceased, inattention, forgetfulness
> - Loss of sense of self or sense of purpose and belonging, feeling aimless or incompetent
> - Feeling disconnected from other people

> Emergence from grief is characterized by the following:
> - Comprehension of the reality and consequences of the death
> - Emergence of positive emotions or memories
> - Thoughts and memories of the deceased are accessible but not preoccupying
> - Restoration of sense of self and sense of purpose and belonging; feelings of competence and well-being
> - Interest and engagement in life and other relationships

**How can you help someone like Betty overcome grief?**
- Utilizing a person's natural support system is important for overcoming grief.
- Additional peer or faith-based support can be helpful. Many health care systems, senior centers, and faith-based agencies offer individual and group-based support services for grief.
- Some patients may benefit from referral to a grief counselor.
- Trusted clinicians can also help patients to accept the reality of the death, gradually confront reminders of the deceased loved one, and start to consider what they want for their future.
- Treatment for the physical symptoms of grief should emphasize self-care and maintaining a healthy lifestyle. Management of sleep disturbances should focus on addressing sleep hygiene and avoidance of sedatives or hypnotics [11].

> **Case 2 (Continued)**
> You learn that Betty has excellent support from her family and her faith community. You make a plan for her to return in 6 months to recheck her diabetes

> and see how she is doing. When she returns to clinic 6 months later and you ask how she is doing, she says, "I don't feel right. I miss my husband every day. Nothing is the same without him." She breaks down in tears. You ask her more about how she has been coping. You find that she has stopped going to church and is no longer getting together with her friends for coffee because these activities remind her of her husband. She finds it too painful to do things that she and her husband used to do together.
>
> You are concerned about the severity of her ongoing symptoms. You step out and ask her to complete the Brief Grief Questionnaire [12]. She scores a 9 (>4 is positive). Further screening for complicated grief and depression is indicated so you ask her to complete the Inventory of Complicated Grief [13].

**How would you distinguish complicated grief from normal or acute grief?**
Complicated grief is a condition that is recognized by many experts; however, the terminology and diagnostic criteria for complicated grief are not well defined.
- DSM-5 [5] includes *provisional* criteria for the diagnosis of "Persistent Complex Bereavement Disorder" (PCBD) defined as a "severe and persistent grief and mourning reaction" based on criteria set by expert consensus.
- ICD11 [14] includes a new diagnosis of "Prolonged Grief Disorder," defined as a "persistent and pervasive grief response characterized by longing for the deceased or persistent preoccupation with the deceased accompanied by intense emotional pain (e.g. sadness, guilt, anger, denial, blame, difficulty accepting the death, feeling one has lost a part of one's self, an inability to experience positive mood, emotional numbness, difficulty in engaging with social or other activities)."

> Features of complicated grief
>
> - Estimated to affect 2–3% of the population worldwide.
> - Risk factors include the following:
>   - Female
>   - Age > 60
>   - Loss of a child or partner
>   - Sudden death of a loved one by violent means
>   - History of mood or anxiety disorders
>   - History of substance use disorder
>   - Multiple recent losses

- Impairs function and is unusually severe and prolonged (minimum of 6 months).
- Characterized by persistent preoccupation with the deceased and inability to accept the loss or imagine a future without the deceased person.
- May include dysfunctional behaviors such as avoiding people, places, or activities that hold reminders of the person or trying to feel close to the person by excessively looking at pictures, listening to recordings of their voice, smelling clothes.

It is also important to distinguish between complicated grief, depression, and PTSD (Table 4.5).

## What treatment options are available for complicated grief?
Psychotherapy

- Psychotherapy has been shown to be effective for managing complicated grief and is considered first-line treatment.
- A short-term approach called complicated grief treatment that typically consists of 16 weekly sessions has been the most well-studied [15].
- Interventions that focus on strategies to target avoidance of thoughts or reminders of the loss have been shown to be most effective [10].

**Table 4.5** Distinguishing complicated grief, major depression, and post-traumatic stress disorder (PTSD)

| Symptoms | Complicated grief | Major depressive disorder | PTSD |
|---|---|---|---|
| Depressed mood | +++ | +++ | + |
| Anhedonia (loss of interest or pleasure) | − | +++ | + |
| Anxiety | + | + | +++ |
| Yearning or longing | +++ | − | − |
| Guilt | ++ | ++ | + |
| Difficulty concentrating | + | ++ | ++ |
| Preoccupying thoughts | ++ | + | +++ |
| Suicidal ideation | ++ | ++ | ++ |
| Change in appetite/eating behaviors | +++ | +++ | − |
| Sleep disturbance | + | +++ | +++ |
| Nightmares | − | + | +++ |

*Source*: Adapted from Shear [10]
+++ diagnostic criterion
++ usually present
+ may be present
− usually not present

Pharmacotherapy

- The combination of psychotherapy and antidepressants has been shown to be more effective than either approach alone [16].
- Pharmacotherapy data are limited. The same principles of pharmacotherapy for depression apply to grief in older adults. Escitalopram and paroxetine have been studied in small, open-label trials and shown to be effective [17]; however, paroxetine is not recommended for older adults due to side effects.
- Benzodiazepines have not been shown to be effective. Short-term hypnotics have not been well-studied in this population and should be used with extreme caution.

> **Case 2 (Continued)**
> After discussing treatment options, Betty agrees to meet with a behavioral health clinician and start low-dose escitalopram. She also decides to start attending a weekly grief support group and starts attending church again.

## References

1. Beekman AT, Copeland JR, Prince MJ. Review of community prevalence of depression in later life. Br J Psychiatry. 1999;174:307–11.
2. Kok RM, Reynolds CF 3rd. Management of depression in older adults: a review. JAMA. 2017;317(20):2114–22.
3. Kessler RC, Berglund P, Demler O, et al. The epidemiology of major depressive disorder: results from the National Comorbidity Survey Replication (NCS-R). JAMA. 2003;289(23):3095–105.
4. Casey DA. Depression in older adults: a treatable medical condition. Prim Care. 2017;44(3):499–510.
5. American Psychiatric Association. Diagnostic and statistical manual of mental disorder. 5th ed. Washington, DC: American Psychiatric Association; 2013.
6. Gaddey HL, Holder K. Unintentional weight loss in older adults. Am Fam Physician. 2014;89(9):718–22.
7. Lexicomp Online. Wolters Kluwer Clinical Drug Information, Inc. Accessed 30 Nov 2019.
8. By the American Geriatrics Society Beers Criteria Update Expert P. American Geriatrics Society 2019 Updated AGS Beers Criteria(R) for potentially inappropriate medication use in older adults. J Am Geriatr Soc. 2019;67(4):674–94.
9. O'Mahony D, O'Sullivan D, Byrne S, O'Connor MN, Ryan C, Gallagher P. STOPP/START criteria for potentially inappropriate prescribing in older people: version 2. Age Ageing. 2015;44(2):213–8.
10. Shear MK. Clinical practice: complicated grief. N Engl J Med. 2015;372(2):153–6.
11. Shear MK, Muldberg S, Periyakoil V. Supporting patients who are bereaved. BMJ. 2017;358:j2854. https://doi.org/10.1136/bmj.j2854.
12. Ito M, Nakajima S, Fujisawa D, et al. Brief measure of screening complicated grief: reliability and discriminant validity. PLoS One. 2012;7(2):e31202. https://doi.org/10.1371/journal.pone.0031209.
13. Prigerson HG, Maciejewski PK, Reynolds CF III, et al. Inventory of complicated grief: a scale to measure maladaptive symptoms of loss. Psychiatry Res. 1995;59(1–2):65–79.
14. ICD-11. Lancet. 2019;393(10188):2275.
15. Shear MK, Frank E, Houck PR, et al. Treatment of complicated grief: a randomized controlled trial. JAMA. 2005;293(21):2601–8.
16. Simon NM, Shear MK, Fagiolini A, et al. Impact of concurrent naturalistic pharmacotherapy on psychotherapy of complicated grief. Psychiatry Res. 2008;159:31–6.
17. Simon NM. Treating complicated grief. JAMA. 2013;310(4):416–23.

# Caring for Caregivers

**5**

Kendra D. Sheppard

> **Key Points**
> 1. Women are the primary caregivers for family members.
> 2. Approximately 25% of caregivers serve for 5 years or more.
> 3. The more help a loved one needs, the more hours a caregiver serves.
> 4. Caregivers self-report fair or poor health in higher numbers than the general population.
> 5. Caregiver burden is common but preventable, and there are screening tools available for clinicians to evaluate.

> **Case**
> Jackie, aged 75, has been the main caregiver for her husband since his stroke 2 years ago. Today, she presents to the clinic for a blood pressure check. Her blood pressure is elevated. You note in the chart that she has not seen you in a year. When you ask how she is doing, she bursts into tears.

A caregiver is a person who provides unpaid care for a dependent child or adult. According to the American Association of Retired Persons (AARP) Public Policy Institute's report, *Caregiving in the United States* [1],

- An estimated 43.5 million adults in the United States have provided unpaid care to an adult or child in the prior 12 months.
- On average, caregivers are mostly women (60%) and approximately 49 years old.

---

K. D. Sheppard (✉)
Sheppard Consulting Services, LLC, Birmingham, AL, USA
e-mail: ksheppard@sheppardconsulting.org

© Springer Nature Switzerland AG 2021
H. W. Brown et al. (eds.), *Challenges in Older Women's Health*,
https://doi.org/10.1007/978-3-030-59058-1_5

- The recipients of their caregiving are also most often women who are approximately 69 years old.
- Twenty-four percent of caregivers serve for 5 years or more.

> **Case (Continued)**
> After Jackie has stopped crying, you ask her again how she has been doing. She states that she has been overwhelmed taking care of her husband. He is requiring help with bathing and dressing and his medicines are very complicated. Additionally, she is managing their finances, which was always his primary responsibility.

**What Do Caregivers Do?** [2]
1. *Assist with basic activities of daily living*: bathing and grooming, dressing, toileting, and transferring from car or shower
2. *Assist with instrumental activities of daily living*: preparing meals, shopping, housekeeping, laundry, finances, medication oversight, and transportation assistance
3. *Attend doctor visits*: Make and attend appointments
4. *Provide emotional support*: Serve as primary companion and supporting both spiritual and emotional needs (not just medical)
5. *Provide back-up care (or respite) services*: Often siblings or children will provide a break to the primary caregiver

Approximately 1 in 3 caregivers use paid caregiving services. Use of paid help is more common among caregivers who are less physically present (long distance or currently employed) and among those whose care recipient's condition has a presumed need for more help with daily activities (such as Alzheimer's disease) [1].

Care recipients of caregivers employed full time are as follows [3]:
- Less likely to receive large amounts of care from their caregivers
- More likely to receive personal care from paid care providers
- More likely to use community services
- More likely to experience service problems than care recipients of non-employed caregivers

Many caregivers report not being comfortable with medical/nursing tasks. The AARP public policy institute published a series of "How-To" videos and resource guides for family caregivers about specific medical/nursing tasks—including preparing special diets, managing incontinence, wound care, mobility, and managing medications. https://www.aarp.org/ppi/initiatives/home-alone-alliance/

> **Case (Continued)**
> Jackie is exhibiting symptoms of caregiver burnout. You ask her to fill out a caregiver stress self-assessment form which comes back positive.

There are several scales available to measure caregiver stress. The Caregiver Self-Assessment Questionnaire was developed by the American Medical Association specifically for doctors to use in the clinic setting. It is available both online and in a pdf format for printing (https://www.healthinaging.org/tools-and-tips/caregiver-self-assessment-questionnaire) and generates a scale that suggests caregiver-related distress. The American Psychological Association has a website with several other self-assessments, including the Zarit Burden Interview (https://www.apa.org/pi/about/publications/caregivers/practice-settings/assessment/tools/stress-burden).

Caregiving can adversely affect the caregivers' mental and physical health [6]. Caregivers self-report worse physical health and have an increased risk of premature death. They also have increased rates of depression and anxiety and use more medication than noncaregivers.

> In the AARP's Public Policy Report, over half (53%) of caregivers indicate that a decline in their health compromises their ability to provide care.

Caregiver stress or burden may first manifest as a decline in health. Other signs of caregiver stress mimic depressive symptoms are as follows [7]:

- Feeling overwhelmed, alone, isolated, or deserted by others
- Sleeping too much or too little
- Gaining or losing a lot of weight
- Feeling tired most of the time
- Losing interest in activities you used to enjoy
- Becoming easily irritated or angered
- Feeling worried or sad often
- Having headaches or body aches often

Taking steps to relieve caregiver stress helps prevent health problems. Box 5.1 lists several tips to mitigate caregiver stress.

> **Box 5.1 Preventing or Managing Caregiver Stress**
>
> *Suggested Tips from the NIH Office of Women's Health to prevent or manage caregiver stress include*:
>
> - *Support Classes.* Some hospitals offer classes that can teach you how to care for someone with an injury or illness. To find these classes, ask your doctor or call your local Area Agency on Aging.
> - *Community caregiving resources including respite.* Many communities have adult daycare services or respite services to give primary caregivers a break from their caregiving duties.
> - *Help from friends and families.* Make a list of ways others can help you. Let helpers choose what they would like to do. For instance, someone might sit with your care recipient while you do an errand or attend your doctor's appointments.
> - *Join a support group.* The Family Caregiver Alliance is just one source to find a caregiver support group (not disease specific) or a group with caregivers (specifically caring for those with the same illness or disability as your loved one). These groups offer a safe space to share stories, pick-up caregiving tips, and get support from the other facing the same challenges as you.
> - *Get and stay organized.* A daily routine is helpful for both the caregiver and the care recipient.
> - *Take time for yourself.* Continue to maintain your hobbies, rest, and stay connected with family and friends.
> - *Maintain your health.* This means choosing to be physically active, eating healthy foods, and getting restful sleep.
> - *Get regular checkups from your doctor.* Share with the physician/nurse team that you are a doctor. Be up front with any symptoms that you are having.
> - *Take a break.* Caring for someone can be overwhelming. Consider taking a break from your job. Under the federal Family and Medical Leave Act, eligible employees can take up to 12 weeks of unpaid leave per year to care for relatives. Companies are beginning to also provide time for caregiving. Ask about your options from your human resources office.

The U.S. Department of Veterans Affairs has a dedicated website for caregiver support (www.caregiver.va.gov). On this site, you will find a caregiver support line, how to contact your local caregiver support coordinator, and a wealth of resources related to caregiving support.

For nonveterans, caregiver support resources can be found via other governmental agencies, nonprofit organizations, and organizations related by chronic condition.

In an office visit, it is possible to bill for care related to caregiver support. Table 5.1 lists several ICD-10 codes.

**Table 5.1** ICD-10 codes related to caring for caregivers

| Code | Definition |
|---|---|
| Z63.6 | Dependent relative needing care at home |
| Z74.8 | Other problems related to care provider dependency |
| Z63.8 | Other specified problems related to primary support group |
| V61.49 | Cares for dependent relative at home |

**Did You Know?**

In 2000, the United States designated November as *National Family Caregivers Month* to honor the 40 million informal caregivers who take care of aging parents, ill spouses, or other loved ones with disabilities who remain at home.

**Table 5.2** Resources for caregivers

| Resource | Organization/website |
|---|---|
| AARP Home and Family Caregiving Resource Center | https://www.aarp.org/caregiving/ |
| Alzheimer's Association online tools page | https://www.alz.org/help-support/resources/online-tools |
| American Cancer Society Caregivers and Family page | https://www.cancer.org/treatment/caregivers/caregiver-resource-guide.html |
| American Heart Association Support Network | https://supportnetwork.heart.org/ |
| Area Agency on Aging | https://www.n4a.org/caregivers |
| Eldercare Locator | https://www.n4a.org/eldercarelocator |
| Family Caregiver Alliance | https://www.caregiver.org/ |
| AGS Health in Aging | https://www.healthinaging.org/tools-and-tips |
| National Academy of Elder Law Attorneys | https://www.naela.org/ |
| National Alliance for Caregiving | https://www.caregiving.org/ |
| Rosalynn Carter Institute for Caregiving | https://www.rosalynncarter.org/ |
| SAGE National Resource Center Caregiving Resource Page | https://www.sageusa.org/resource-category/caregiving/ |

**Case (Continued)**

You talk to Jackie about her stress. You emphasize that it is common for caregivers to need more support and gently remind her that if she lets her own health suffer, she will not be able to care for her husband. You refer her to community resources (Table 5.2) so that she can get some help at home and maybe respite care. You schedule a follow-up visit to see her in a month and also refer her to your social worker to help her connect with community resources.

## References

1. Caregiving in the US. AARP Public Policy Institute.
2. Caregiving Duties and Responsibilities Guide. https://www.vantagemobility.com/blog/caregiver-duties-responsibilities-home-care; Accessed 1 Nov 2019.
3. Scharlach AE, Gustavson K, Dal Santo TS. Assistance received by employed caregivers and their care recipients: who helps care recipients when caregivers work full time? Gerontologist. 2007;47(6):752–62. https://doi.org/10.1093/geront/47.6.752.
4. https://www.aarp.org/ppi/initiatives/home-alone-alliance/
5. Levine C, Reinhard SC. "It all falls on me" Family caregiver perspectives on medication management, wound care, and video instruction. September 2016 AARP Public Policy Institute Spotlight 22.
6. https://www.cdc.gov/aging/caregiving/index.htm; Content source: Division of Population Health, National Center for Chronic Disease Prevention and Health Promotion
7. https://www.womenshealth.gov/a-z-topics/caregiver-stress
8. https://www.caregiver.va.gov/
9. https://www.healthinaging.org/tools-and-tips/caregiver-self-assessment-questionnaire

# Cancer Survivorship in Women 65 Years and Older

James E. Haine, Noelle K. LoConte, and Amye J. Tevaarwerk

**Key Points**
1. A cancer survivor is "any person with a history of cancer, from the time of diagnosis through the remainder of life." Thus, the term "survivor" includes patients treated with both curative and palliative intent.
2. The number of cancer survivors in the United States exceeds 16 million and the estimated number of survivors treated with curative versus palliative intent is not entirely understood. However, most survivors are expected to live 5 or more years past diagnosis, many with chronic needs related to cancer diagnosis as well as higher rates of comorbid chronic health conditions.
3. Cancer-related information that should be easily available in patients' charts includes cancer type, stage, past treatment, complications of past treatment, and plans for ongoing cancer-related care. This may be

J. E. Haine (✉)
Division of General Internal Medicine, Department of Internal Medicine,
University of Wisconsin School of Medicine and Public Health, Madison, WI, USA
e-mail: james.haine@uwmf.wisc.edu

N. K. LoConte
Department of Medicine, University of Wisconsin Carbone Cancer Center,
University of Wisconsin School of Medicine and Public Health, Madison, WI, USA
e-mail: ns3@medicine.wisc.edu

A. J. Tevaarwerk
Division of Hematology, Oncology and Palliative Care, Department of Medicine,
University of Wisconsin Carbone Cancer Center, University of Wisconsin School of Medicine and Public Health, Madison, WI, USA
e-mail: at4@medicine.wisc.edu

> provided to patients by oncology clinicians as a treatment summary and/or a survivorship care plan, which may act as tools for communication, collaboration, and care coordination.
> 4. Common preventative health interventions such as maintaining positive energy balance through diet and exercise, quitting tobacco, and reducing alcohol can reduce the risk of cancer recurrence, death, and all-cause mortality in cancer survivors.
> 5. Common long-term adverse effects of cancer and cancer-related treatments are likely to be encountered and treated by nononcology clinicians.

## Introduction

The term "cancer survivor" is now widely agreed upon as "any person with a history of cancer, from the time of diagnosis through the remainder of life" [1, 2]. This definition encompasses a wide range of experiences and includes the time of diagnosis, periods of treatment, cancer-free survival, chronic or intermittent disease, and end-of-life care. The term "cancer survivor" does not necessarily imply that a patient was treated with curative intent. However, most patients at very high risk for recurrence or with advanced/metastatic disease are followed continuously by their cancer care team. Survivors treated with curative intent, particularly those with lower risk of recurrence or at some distance from diagnosis, may be discharged to primary care or have their care shared between primary care and other specialties, although models and standards for follow-up care vary widely [3].

> **Most Prevalent Cancers in US Women >65 [1]**
> 1. Breast cancer
> 2. Colorectal cancer
> 3. Uterine cancer

Therefore, for this overview of cancer survivorship in women over age 65, we will focus on patients without metastatic cancer that have transitioned from active cancer treatment to extended and long-term survival from their cancer. The number of cancer survivors in the United States has increased from approximately 3.6 million in 1975 to an estimated 16.9 million as of January 1, 2019 and is projected to exceed 22 million by 2030 based on the growth and aging of the US population alone [1, 4]. Of these estimated 16.9 million survivors, roughly 8.8 million are women and over 5.2 million are aged 65 or older. With the aging of the baby boomers and consequent increasing incidence of cancer, the average age of cancer survivors is expected to continue rising in the next decade [5]. Nearly half of these female cancer survivors were diagnosed with breast cancer. Solid tumors of adult-onset (e.g., breast, colon) vastly outnumber hematologic malignancies (e.g., leukemia, lymphoma) [1], but hematologic malignancy survivors have significant differences in treatment and thus late and long-term effects.

> *Late or future effect*: Often rare, late side effects cancer treatment may only develop in the (distant) future (e.g., second cancers from radiation).

> *Long-term or chronic effect*: These typically develop on or shortly after treatment, and then persist life-long (e.g., neuropathy from chemotherapy).

In addition to late and long-term effects from cancer and/or cancer treatments, rates of comorbid health conditions are higher in cancer survivors compared with patients without a history of cancer (54% vs. 45%, respectively) [6]. Follow-up with primary care is central to ensuring appropriate care for comorbid conditions [7]. Common long-term adverse effects of cancer and cancer-related treatments are also likely to be encountered and treated by primary care providers (PCPs) [8]. Finally, shortages of both primary and oncology physicians are predicted in the near future [9, 10] increasing the need to better coordinate and shared care for survivors in order to meet essential components of high-quality cancer survivorship care [11].

> **Essential Components of Cancer Survivorship**
> 1. Prevention
> 2. Surveillance
> 3. Intervention
> 4. Coordination

The essential components of cancer survivorship care were defined in the 2000s, and emphasize a combination of screening for recurrence or late effects, and managing persistent late and long-term effects [2]. For example, a cancer follow-up visit for a patient with Stage III colorectal cancer who is a few years out from diagnosis and treatment might include the following:

- *Prevention* of recurrence and new cancers by ensuring that the patient is taking aspirin daily.
- *Surveillance* for late psychosocial effects such as depression.
- *Intervention* with management for oxaliplatin-induced neuropathy.
- *Coordination* of follow-up colonoscopy.

Emphasis has been placed on attempting to coordinate this care with primary care, including either sharing or transitioning this care entirely to PCPs as appropriate. Practically speaking, what this looks like varies a great deal from region

> **Case**
>
> You are meeting "Barbara" for the first time at an office visit. She is a 70-year-old woman who has recently moved to the area to live closer to children. She needs a new primary care provider. She is able to tell you that she has a history of left-sided breast cancer diagnosed 3 years ago, and that she had surgery, chemotherapy, and radiation. She is taking anastrozole and needs a refill of this.
>
> She notes that she has ongoing hot flashes, recurrent difficulty with left arm swelling, vaginal dryness and pain, and moderate burning and tingling in both feet since cancer treatment that she indicates are bothersome to her daily life. PHQ 9 and GAD 7 screening scores are both elevated at 12.

**Table 6.1** Brief guide to available online resources

| | |
|---|---|
| The American Society of Clinical Oncology (ASCO). Both ASCO.org and Cancer.net have specific survivorship sections. | ASCO.org<br>Patient-facing: Cancer.net |
| The National Comprehensive Cancer Network (NCCN) has both patient and clinician facing informational sites each with specific survivorship sections. | NCCN.org<br>It is free to create a login—You don't have to be a member, but you do need an account. |
| The American Cancer Society (ACS) website for patient and clinician resources. ACS also has a survivorship app available for iPhone (but not currently available for other operating systems) with FAQ in survivorship care. | cancer.org<br>cancer.org/health-care-professionals<br>FAQ: https://www.cancer.org/health-care-professionals/national-cancer-survivorship-resource-center/survivorship-guidlines-app-faq.html |
| The Centers for Disease Control and Prevention (CDC) has cancer informational resources for both patients and clinicians including specific survivorship sections. | CDC.gov/cancer |
| The National Cancer Survivorship Resource Center at the George Washington University Cancer center. This includes clinician and patient toolkits as well as a cancer survivorship eLearning series for primary care providers. | https://smhs.gwu.edu/gwci/survivorship/ncsrc |

to region, clinic to clinic, provider to provider, and patient to patient. *This heterogeneity is among the most challenging aspects of cancer survivorship.*

A plethora of resources exist online, and like the internet in general, some are well-vetted than others. Listed in the table below are common, widely used, and freely available resources that we recommend to providers, although some also have patient-facing information. For specific cancer types, guidelines may exist with specific follow-up recommendations, which are updated periodically (Table 6.1).

**What Cancer-Related Information Is Important for PCPs to Have on Hand?** Keeping the above case study in mind, we've attempted to outline the general cancer-related information that is helpful for PCPs to have available.

- *What is the diagnosis?* What type of cancer, and what was the stage? Are there any available receptors or markers on pathology that affect prognosis and treatment?
    - This information can generally be located in oncology notes, pathology reports, and survivorship care plans.
    - There are many cancer staging systems. Cancer staging systems may be specific to certain cancer types. The most widely used for solid tumors is the TNM staging system. This includes information listing the tumor location and cell type (i.e., pancreatic adenocarcinoma). This is followed by staging of primary tumor size and possible invasion of adjacent structures (T0–4), number and location of involved lymph nodes (N0–4), and whether or not the cancer has metastasized (M0–1). An "X" rather than number means primary tumor, lymph node involvement, or metastatic disease that cannot be measured or has not been assessed. M1 typically (but not always) indicates metastatic disease for which treatment is not curative but may be life prolonging or for palliation of symptoms.
    - Additional information that may be reported includes tumor grade and receptors or markers specific to different types of cancer.
    - For instance, in breast cancer cases diagnosed 2012–2016, approximately 77% of tumors express estrogen receptors (ER) and progesterone receptors (PR), 14% overexpress human epidermal growth factor receptor 2 (HER 2), approximately 14% are "triple negative" (meaning negative for ER, PR, and HER 2), and 8% are receptor status unknown [12]. Expression of all, some, or none of these is important to know when deciding treatment and communicating with oncology providers.
    - Hematologic malignancies such as leukemia, lymphoma, and myeloma have disease-specific staging systems.
- *What cancer-related treatment has been rendered?* What are the possible complications of cancer or cancer-related treatment? The treatments used, in combination with patient health and age, determine the specific complications likely to be faced. Hematologic cancers are typically treated primarily with systemic therapies. Solid tumors, by contrast, are typically treated with both local and systemic options, unless the risk of metastatic recurrence is low and/or the patient is not expected to benefit (e.g., life expectancy and frailty).
    - Surgery and radiation tend to cause localized side effects to the site of treatment (e.g., fibrosis and lymphedema).
    - Medical therapies (chemotherapy, targeted therapy, etc.) can cause systemic side effects (e.g., peripheral neuropathy and osteoporosis).

- *Is treatment ongoing?* If treatment is ongoing, what future treatments are planned, what is the proposed end date? What is the planned monitoring and/or possible complications?
    - It is not unreasonable to revisit the need for monitoring for recurrence or new primaries as survivors develop other life-limiting illnesses or as they advance in age. However, because this typically varies based on type and stage of cancer, it is likely best to do so after touching base with the oncology clinic or cancer care team.
- *Was genetic testing done?* Has any genetic testing been done or been recommended to assess for inheritable (germline) conditions?
    - Family history changes over time, as do genetic testing guidelines! New information may arise that is concerning for inherited cancer syndrome, and patients that did not meet criteria for genetic testing in the past may now meet them. Patients with histories concerning for an inherited cancer syndrome should be referred for genetic counseling prior to testing.
    - This includes considering updated recommendations for patients who are more distant from diagnosis. Current guidelines for ovarian and pancreatic patients indicate that all patients should be tested, regardless of family history. This applies to patients who have been discharged from oncology and may only follow with a PCP.

> **Possible Treatment Modalities**
> *Local*
> - Surgery, including organ transplant
> - Radiation
> - Interventional procedures
>
> *Systemic*
> - Cytotoxic chemotherapy, including hematologic stem cell transplants
> - Targeted therapy, including HER2, and small-molecule tyrosine kinase inhibitors
> - Endocrine therapy
> - Immunotherapy

**Survivorship Care Plans** Survivorship care plans have been recommended to improve communication among oncology specialists, patients, and primary care providers. Survivorship care plans are typically patient-centered documents that include a summary of information recommended above plus additional recommendations for improving overall health. These are typically provided to survivors at

> **Key Points**
> 1. Local therapies typically address spread of the cancer in a region, and may prevent a local recurrence. Systemic therapies typically address the risk of widespread or metastatic recurrence.
> 2. Hematologic cancers are typically treated with systemic therapies. Solid tumors, by contrast, are typically treated with both local and systemic options.
> 3. Revisit the need for monitoring for recurrence with the patient's oncology team.
> 4. Periodically review need for genetic testing.

the end of active treatment (e.g., surgery, chemotherapy, and/or radiation) and *not* at the time of discharge from oncology. There is great variability surrounding their use in the oncology community. However, if available, a survivorship care plan should contain all of the recommended cancer-related diagnosis and treatment history.

> **Case (Continued)**
> You find and document her cancer stage (Stage Ib), receptor status (ER+ PR+ HER2-), past surgery (lumpectomy with sentinel lymph node removal), radiation therapy completed, and chemotherapy (TC or Taxotere/Cytoxan).
>
> Her PHQ—9 and GAD 7 scores indicate possible anxiety and/or depression present that can be explored and possibly treated further. She has likely lymphedema and peripheral neuropathy related to past cancer treatment that can be ameliorated. She walks 30 min daily and asks what over-the-counter supplements will help her fight cancer.
>
> She wonders if she can receive a flu shot while taking anastrozole.

**What Are Common Cancer Survivorship Issues That PCPs Are Likely to Encounter?** Keeping the case study in mind, we've attempted to outline the general cancer-related issues that are likely to arise in the primary care clinic and may be best addressed there.

- *Many cancer survivors have questions about the impact of healthy lifestyle choices.* Promoting healthy lifestyle choices such as quitting smoking, minimizing or ceasing alcohol, and maintaining positive energy balance through diet and exercise as key components of cancer survivorship is crucial.
  - Quitting smoking or other tobacco use is recommended by the American Cancer Society (ACS) for everyone.

- The ACS has guidelines on nutrition and exercise for cancer survivors [13]: https://www.cancer.org/healthy/eat-healthy-get-active/acs-guidelines-nutrition-physical-activity-cancer-prevention/guidelines.html
- A brief summary of the guidelines includes the following:
    1. Maintain a healthy weight. If overweight, even a small amount of weight loss can have benefits.
    2. Weekly exercise goal of 150 min of moderate intensity or 75 min of vigorous intensity exercise preferably spread throughout the week.
    3. Healthy diet with five or more servings of fruits and vegetables per day and limited amount of red meats and processed foods.
    4. Limit alcohol intake to no more than one drink per day for women and two drinks per day for men.

- *Safety and timing of vaccinations are frequently the subject of questions.* Per 2014 NCCN guideline [14]:
    - Vaccination of *solid tumor* cancer survivors is encouraged, and can generally follow the usual schedule for other patients of similar age and health status as long as they are not actively immunosuppressed (e.g., on cytotoxic chemotherapy).
        1. *Inactivated influenza vaccine is encouraged.* Administration >2 weeks before or >3 months after completion of chemotherapy is preferred due to better immune response. However, influenza vaccine can be administered during cancer treatment, if necessary. Vaccination of caregivers and close contacts is also encouraged.
        2. Other inactivated or recombinant vaccines should be administered >2 weeks before cancer treatment and >3 months after cancer chemotherapy.
        3. Live vaccines are contraindicated in actively immune-suppressed patients and should be given >4 weeks before or >3 months after completion of cancer chemotherapy. Consultation with oncology or other providers experienced in vaccination of patients with cancer is encouraged prior to administration of live vaccines.
    - Vaccination of *hematologic* cancer survivors is likewise encouraged, but can be more nuanced, especially if the survivor has undergone hematologic stem cell transplant (also known as bone marrow transplant, whether autologous or allogenic).
        1. In survivors who have received anti-B-cell antibody treatment (i.e., Rituximab), vaccinations other than inactivated influenza should be delayed for at least 6 months after last dose of such therapy.
        2. For patients who have received a stem cell transplant (whether autologous or allogenic), the treating Transplant Center should be consulted or may have provided specific recommendations.

- *Many cancer survivors utilize complementary and alternative medicines and treatments* [15].
  - Like many other Americans, cancer survivors often access complementary and alternative medications and treatments to treat either cancer or cancer treatment side effects. Asking about the use is an important aspect of history. The NIH National Center for Complementary and Integrative Health has an excellent online resource to provide additional information and help answer patient and clinician questions: https://smhs.gwu.edu/gwci/survivorship/ncsrc
- *Fear of cancer recurrence is a significant and common concern among cancer survivors* [16].
  - Fear of cancer recurrence is not strongly linked with prognosis and may occur in patients despite a relatively good prognosis [17].
  - Clinicians should reinforce that fear of recurrence is common, normal, and may be helpful if it leads to increased commitment to making healthy lifestyle choices and following through with recommended follow-up [18].
  - However, if fear of recurrence is significant and distressing, intervention with health psychology can be beneficial [17].
  - Information to help patients cope with fear of recurrence can be found at Cancer.net—https://www.cancer.net/survivorship/life-after-cancer/coping-with-fear-recurrence
- *Symptoms of anxiety and depression are common in cancer survivors* [19].
  - As with other cases of anxiety and depression, treatment with cognitive behavioral therapy, mindfulness-based stress reduction, physical activity, and medication such as SSRI, SNRI, and gabapentin can be beneficial [19].
  - Gabapentin or SNRI may also help other symptoms such as hot flashes and peripheral neuropathy [19].
- *Fatigue in cancer survivors may have more than one cause.*
  - Chemotherapy, radiation therapy, and many medications used to treat cancer can cause fatigue, but generally improve over time as survivors recover. Not all survivors will feel that they recover completely to a precancer baseline.
  - Anemia, insomnia, anxiety and depression, and changes in activity and nutrition may also contribute.
  - Treatment of fatigue is aimed at adjusting comorbid medications when possible, treating other underlying disorders if present, and encouraging healthy lifestyle. Moderate exercise, yoga, and psychosocial interventions such as cognitive behavioral therapies, and mindfulness-based therapies are recommended for treatment [20].
  - The 2014 American Society of Clinical Oncology (ASCO) clinical guideline on management of fatigue in cancer survivors can be found at: https://ascopubs.org/doi/abs/10.1200/JCO.2013.53.4495

- *Cancer survivors may complain of post-treatment cognitive impairment*
    - Patients often refer to their symptoms as "Chemo brain" or "Chemo fog". However, while symptoms are more commonly reported in survivors that have received chemotherapy, symptoms are also reported after surgery, radiation (especially, brain radiation), or hormone therapy.
    - Risk factors and etiology are being investigated and are likely multifactorial.
    - Typically, patients will note short-term memory difficulties such as difficulty in remembering a list of items or trouble with word finding. It is very unusual to develop progressive impairment that affects daily function at a substantial level or for the symptoms to progressively worsen over time.

> Forty-five percent of patients with breast cancer report a decline in cognitive function following chemotherapy [21].

- *Post-treatment cognitive impairment is a diagnosis of exclusion. New, severe, or persistent cases should be evaluated for other causes of impairment such as metastatic disease.*
    - Treatment is largely aimed at other underlying disorders if present (e.g., depression and sleep disturbance), and encouraging healthy lifestyle.
- *Sexual dysfunction and low libido are significant concerns for female cancer survivors, particularly those undergoing treatment for breast and pelvic cancers* [22]. *Specific considerations that may apply include the following*:
    - Fatigue, anxiety, depression, and altered body image can contribute to sexual dysfunction and low libido.
    - Vaginal stenosis due to pelvic radiation or surgery can cause vaginal pain and bleeding [23].
    - Endocrine therapy can block or lower systemic estrogen levels and can result in hot flashes, low libido, and atrophic vaginal symptoms [24]. Venlafaxine and less commonly gabapentin can be used to treat hot flashes.
        1. Nonhormonal therapies, including vaginal lubrication, may help dryness (See also Chapter 1).
        2. Risks from systemic absorption of vaginal estrogen may be lower when combined with tamoxifen since tamoxifen blocks estrogen receptor in breast tissue.

    *In patients with breast cancer, it is advisable to touch base with medical oncology before starting a vaginal hormone therapy as safety data are mixed or largely unavailable.*
- *Cancer survivorship can carry a significant financial "toxicity" with effects lasting years after diagnosis and treatment* [25].

– Clinicians should inquire about fiscal and/or insurance burdens and refer patients to social work or other support services available.

> **Case (Continued)**
> You discuss with Barbara that at this point, influenza and all other vaccinations are safe and recommended. She is congratulated on and encouraged to continue regular walking. You discuss concerns about over the counter supplements and give her information to look through from the ACS so that she can make an informed decision about taking them.
> Given her elevated PHQ 9 and GAD 7 scores, you discuss seeing a health psychologist and the possibility of treating her with an antidepressant. Venlafaxine or duloxetine, both SNRIs, may help mood disorders as well as reduce discomfort from peripheral neuropathy and hot flashes (See also Chapter 4).
> On examination, you note mild left arm swelling and multiple telangiectasias on the skin over her left breast.

*Symptoms, late, and long-term effects for cancer survivors are mediated by many factors*. These include host (age, weight, co-morbidities, etc.), cancer location (breast, colon, left vs. right, etc.), and treatment factors (surgery, radiation, medical therapies used, etc.), making it difficult to generalize. Keeping the case study in mind, we have attempted to outline the general site-specific concerns, based on common cancers and treatments typically used in older female survivors.

**Common Issues After Cancer Surgery** Surgery tends to cause local complications, with findings confined to the area operated on. Most long-term and late effects of treatment are caused by scarring and/or abnormal adhesions in the area. Issues include lymphedema (as noted below, radiation is a risk factor for lymphedema as well); scarring including retractions leading to reduced range of motion, abdominal adhesions and fistulas, and changes in organ function (such as diminished lung capacity following lobectomy). Specific concerns for breast and GI survivors include the following:

- *Lymphedema* or abnormal lymphatic fluid collection (pitting or nonpitting) can occur after removal or damage to lymph nodes.
    - Most commonly perceived in an extremity after removal of axillary or pelvic lymph nodes, but may also occur in trunk (breast or chest wall), genitals, or head. The risk increases with the number of nodes removed, radiation therapy to lymph node areas, and obesity.
    - Mainstay of treatment is prompt occupational therapy to supervise manual lymphatic drainage and compression as well as prompt treatment of infection if present.
    - Flares can be prevented by avoiding trauma and weight gain and using compression sleeves as needed.

- *Malabsorption or diarrhea* may result from hemicolectomies for colon cancer, abdominoperineal resection for rectal cancer, or pancreatic insufficiency due to pancreatic resection.

  – Nearly half of all colorectal cancer survivors have chronic diarrhea at completion of treatment [26, 27]. First line treatment for persistent diarrhea following hemicolectomy or abdominoperineal resection includes fiber and antidiarrhea medication such as loperamide or diphenoxylate/atropine. Chronic diarrhea may predispose to fecal incontinence (See also Chapter 11).
  – Pancreatic enzyme replacement may be beneficial in the setting of pancreatic resection.
  – For patients with permanent ostomy placement, significant quality-of-life challenges on physical activity, sexuality and intimacy, travel, and psychological well-being have been reported [28].
  – Potential ostomy-related complications include skin conditions, hernia and fistula formation, and urinary retention.

> **Common Persistent Issues After Surgery**
> - Lymphedema
> - Scarring, adhesions, and fistulas
> - Diminished organ function

> **Case (Continued)**
> Barbara appears to have ongoing difficulty with lymphedema in her left arm due to her cancer surgery and radiation. She is offered occupational therapy referral.

**Common Issues After Cancer Radiation** Radiation tends to cause local complications, with findings confined to the field irradiated. Most long-term and late effects of radiation treatment are due to tissue fibrosis in the radiation field. The risk of long-term effects from radiation is typically based on techniques developed decades ago, and may not reflect the likelihood with more modern radiation techniques. Issues include lymphedema; scarring including retractions, abdominal adhesions, and lung fibrosis; fistulas; and skin discoloration and/or telangiectasias. Radiation can also result in second cancers, such as sarcomas, squamous cell and basal cancer, and fragile bones within a radiation field. *Specific concerns for Breast, GI, and Gyn survivors include the following*:

- *Range of motion* changes due to scarring and retraction over the chest wall.
- *Vaginal stenosis* can cause dyspareunia and postcoital bleeding. A pelvic exam is highly recommended to exclude malignant cause of symptoms but should be

carried out by an experienced clinician. Vaginal dilators are commonly used to treat stenosis, although evidence of benefit is lacking. Other optimal topical treatments and hormone replacement also require additional study [23]. Pelvic floor physical therapy may also be beneficial for dyspareunia [44].
- *Radiation cystitis* can vary in severity and may cause hematuria, suprapubic pain, urinary frequency, urgency, dysuria, and increased risk of infection. Bladder infection and malignancy should be ruled out. Treatment can include anticholinergic medications for mild cases or urologic intervention for moderate-to-severe symptoms [29]. Pelvic floor physical therapy may also be beneficial [44].
- *Chronic radiation proctitis (CRP)* occurs in 5–10% of patients that receive pelvic radiation. Presenting symptoms include rectal bleeding, fecal urgency, diarrhea, and mucous discharge. Endoscopy is needed to evaluate for malignancy, stricture, and the extent of radiation-induced disease. Mild CRP with minimal bleeding can be treated with loperamide, fiber, stool bulking agents, and topical steroids [29]. These patients may also be predisposed to fecal incontinence (See also Chapter 11).

**Common Persistent Issues After Radiation**
- Lymphedema
- Scarring, adhesions, and fistulas
- Skin discoloration

Radiation to the *central* or *left* chest wall can potentially increase the risk of cardiovascular disease because the heart may be included in the field. Increased rates of coronary artery disease, valvular heart disease, conduction abnormalities, restrictive cardiomyopathy with heart failure, and constrictive pericarditis have been observed but this risk typically takes years to develop [33]. Consensus guidelines on screening patients for cardiac disease after chest radiation are lacking, especially for older adults.

**Case (Continued)**
Barbara is reassured that skin telangiectasias following radiation therapy are benign. She is examined for skin cancer.

**Common Late and Long-Term Issues After Medical Therapy** In contrast to surgery and radiation, medical therapies for cancer can cause systemic side effects. Medical therapies currently include a broad and ever-expanding list of options. Common chemotherapies that would be used in older female survivors include doxorubicin, paclitaxel or docetaxel, and cyclophosphamide in breast cancer; 5-fluoruracil and oxaliplatin in colorectal cancer; and paclitaxel and cisplatin or carboplatin in gynecologic cancers.

> **Types of Medical Therapy**
> - Cytotoxic chemotherapy
> - Endocrine therapy
> - Immunotherapy
> - Targeted antibody

- *Peripheral neuropathy* is common although incidence varies based on chemotherapy drug used, dose, and duration [30]. The drugs with the highest incidence are platinum agents (cisplatin, carboplatin, or oxaliplatin), taxanes (paclitaxel or docetaxel), vinca alkaloids, and bortezomib.
    - Chemotherapy-induced peripheral neuropathy is predominantly sensory rather than motor or autonomic and presents in a symmetrical "stocking-glove" distribution.
    - There may be initial worsening of symptoms even after chemotherapy is stopped, then gradual improvement followed by stabilization of symptoms. *Peripheral neuropathy that appears more than 6 months after completion of therapy is less likely to be due to chemotherapy and alternate explanations should be explored.*
    - Oxaliplatin-related neuropathy is made worse with exposure to cold. The other neuropathies are largely dose-related effects.
    - Physical therapy for patients with gait and mobility limitations may reduce risk of falls [31].
    - For patients with painful chemotherapy-induced peripheral neuropathy, 2014 American Society of Clinic Oncology (ASCO) guidelines recommend trial of duloxetine to treat pain [32].
        1. Other pharmacologic modalities such as gabapentin/pregabalin, tricyclic antidepressants, and a topical compounded gel (ketamine, amitriptyline, and baclofen) do not have evidence to support efficacy but may be tried given lack of other options and benefit in other conditions with neuropathic pain [32].
        2. Small trials show acupuncture may offer benefit, but a systemic review concluded that there is insufficient evidence to recommend it [34]. However, given the low likelihood of harm, trial of acupuncture in a patient who desires it is reasonable.

> **Case (Continued)**
> The trial of duloxetine previously discussed may help with mood hot flashes and peripheral neuropathy. Venlafaxine has more data to support use for hot flashes but not significant data to support use for peripheral neuropathy.

- *Cardiac complications.* Medication-induced damage to heart muscle resulting in systolic congestive heart failure can occur from exposure to many different chemotherapeutic agents.
  - Monoclonal antibodies used to treat many different cancers, such as trastuzumab for HER2-positive cancers (breast as well as other cancers such as esophageal, gastric, and cholangiocarcinomas), can cause reduced ejection fraction during treatment. This is generally reversible with significant recovery possible when treatment is completed.
  - Irreversible cardiac damage, which can become apparent during treatment or late onset, is most commonly associated with anthracycline chemotherapy frequently used in treatment of breast and gynecologic cancers, sarcoma, and lymphoma.
  - ASCO recommends counseling and treatment regarding other modifiable risk factors such as smoking, hypertension, dyslipidemia, diabetes, and obesity to lessen cardiac risk [35].
  - In patients with other risk factors, such as age > 65 with exposure to anthracyclines, an echocardiogram performed 6–12 months after completion of therapy is reasonable. There is no consensus to recommend additional monitoring in asymptomatic individuals, although threshold to evaluate for systolic dysfunction with echocardiogram should be low in patients with symptoms of heart failure [35].
  - Treatment of cancer therapy-related heart failure is similar to that for other forms of chronic systolic congestive heart failure with beta-blockers, ACE-inhibitor or angiotensin receptor blockers, and diuretics. Referral to cardiologist is recommended [35].

For the most part, non-metastatic colorectal and gynecologic cancer survivors do not receive long-term maintenance therapy. However, patients with hormone-receptor positive breast cancer will typically be on an endocrine therapy for 5 or more years. For this reason, we have devoted a little additional time to specific considerations with these agents.

**Endocrine Therapy** Women that have been diagnosed with hormone-receptor positive breast cancer will commonly receive endocrine therapy with tamoxifen or an aromatase inhibitor (anastrozole, letrozole, or exemestane) for a variable duration of 5–10 years.

- *Aromatase inhibitors* (letrozole, anastrozole, and exemestane) block the peripheral conversion of androgens to estrogen to lower estrogen levels below normal post-menopausal levels. They are frequently preferred for cancer treatment in the post-menopausal setting as they are more effective at reducing risk of cancer recurrence than tamoxifen and have a potentially more acceptable safety profile [36].

- Diffuse arthralgia is a common side effect commonly seen within the first few months of starting the medication and tends to affect multiple joints after an individual has been at rest. Switching among AIs is a common practice, but duloxetine and acupuncture may also be options [37].
- Accelerated loss of bone density is also a risk. Regular monitoring for and treatment of osteopenia/osteoporosis is recommended [38]. There is some variance in guidelines on how often to check a bone density test while taking an aromatase inhibitor; typically, bone density testing is recommended every 1–3 years. Medicare will generally not cover checking more often than every 2 years.
- Coronary artery disease is a potential concern based on meta-analysis data [39].

- *Tamoxifen* and *toremifene* are selective estrogen receptor modulator that inhibits growth of breast cancer cells by competitive antagonism of the estrogen receptor. Tamoxifen is typically used in the United States.

  - In contrast to aromatase inhibitors, tamoxifen will improve bone density in postmenopausal women, but mildly increases the risk of DVT/PE (2–3×) and endometrial cancer (1/1000/year → 2/1000/year).
  - Guidelines recommend against asymptomatic screening for endometrial cancer on tamoxifen [40], but it is important to inquire regularly about postmenopausal vaginal bleeding and arrange prompt evaluation for endometrial biopsy in women taking tamoxifen.
  - Tamoxifen is converted into active form by CYP2D6 and there are potential interactions with inhibitors of this.

    1. Many antidepressants interact with CYP2D6 to reduce active form of tamoxifen. Paroxetine, fluoxetine, and bupropion have the most effect. Citalopram/escitalopram and venlafaxine have the least.
    2. A recent cohort study did not show difference in mortality between patients taking antidepressants that were potent inhibitors of CYP2D6 and those that were not potent inhibitors [41].
    3. In patients already taking tamoxifen, we generally avoid starting one of the potent CYP2D6-inhibiting antidepressants. However, in patients already stable on a potent CYP2D6-inhibiting antidepressant that are starting tamoxifen, we do not require a change in antidepressant.
    4. Tamoxifen also has a significant interaction with warfarin, causing increased INR and risk of bleeding. If they are used together, a dose reduction in warfarin and frequent monitoring are recommended. Other anticoagulant options should be considered when possible.

**Case (Continued)**
Recognizing that Barbara is taking anastrozole, an aromatase inhibitor, you specifically review her history to ensure that she has up-to-date bone density testing every 2 years.

**Monitoring for Cancer Recurrence** Updated evidence-based guidelines on monitoring for cancer recurrence for various cancer types are available at the online resources noted above. If a survivorship care plan is available, it should include recommended follow-up testing. Multiple available reviews show poor adherence to follow-up guidelines in the United States, both by oncologists and PCPs, with a wide variation of over- and under-testing [42, 43].

## Conclusion

The number of cancer survivors in the United States, particularly over age 65, is growing rapidly. Primary care clinicians currently have a key role in promoting quality cancer survivorship care, and this role will likely continue to expand in the upcoming decade based on the increasing number of survivors.

## References

1. Cancer Treatment and Survivorship Facts & Figures 2019–2021. https://www.cancer.org/content/dam/cancer-org/research/cancer-facts-and-statistics/cancer-treatment-and-survivorship-facts-and-figures/cancer-treatment-and-survivorship-facts-and-figures-2019-2021.pdf. Accessed 12 Dec 2019.
2. Hewitt ME, et al. From cancer patient to cancer survivor: lost in transition. Washington, DC: The National Academies Press; 2006. xxv, 506 p.
3. Nekhlyudov L, Omalley DM, Hudson SV. Integrating primary care providers in the care of cancer survivors: gaps in evidence and future opportunities. Lancet Oncol. 2017. https://doi.org/10.1016/s1470-2045(16)30570-8.
4. Miller KD, Noqueira L, Mariotto AB, Rowland JH, Yabroff KR, Alfano CM, et al. Cancer treatment and survivorship statistics, 2019. CA Cancer J Clin. 2019;69(5):363–85.
5. Bluethmann SM, Mariotto AB, Rowland JH. Anticipating the "silver tsunami": prevalence trajectories and comorbidity burden among older cancer survivors in the United States. Cancer Epidemiol Biomark Prev. 2016;25:1029–36.
6. Yabroff KR, Lawrence WF, Clauser S, Davis WW, Brown ML. Burden of illness in Cancer survivors: findings from a population-based National Sample. J Natl Cancer Inst. 2004;96:1322–30.
7. Snyder CF, Frick KD, Herbert RJ, Blackford AL, Neville BA, Lemke KW, Carducci MA, Wolff AC, Earle CC. Comorbid condition care quality in cancer survivors: role of primary care and specialty providers and care coordination. J Cancer Surviv. 2015;9:641–9.
8. Donohue S, et al. Cancer survivorship care plan utilization and impact on clinical decision-making at point-of-care visits with primary care: results from an engineering, primary care, and oncology collaborative for survivorship health. J Cancer Educ. 2019;34(2):252–8.
9. Petterson SM, Liaw WR, Phillips RL, Rabin DL, Meyers DS, Bazemore AW. Projecting US primary care physician workforce needs: 2010-2025. Ann Fam Med. 2012;10:503–9.
10. Shulman LN, Jacobs LA, Greenfield S, et al. Cancer care and Cancer survivorship Care in the United States: will we be able to Care for these Patients in the future? J Oncol Pract. 2009;5:119–23.
11. Moor JSD, Mariotto AB, Parry C, Alfano CM, Padgett L, Kent EE, Forsythe L, Scoppa S, Hachey M, Rowland JH. Cancer survivors in the United States: prevalence across the survivorship trajectory and implications for care. Cancer Epidemiol Biomark Prev. 2013;22:561–70.
12. SEER Cancer Statistics Review, 1975–2016 [Internet]. SEER. [cited 2019 Dec 12]. Available from: https://seer.cancer.gov/csr/1975_2016/

13. Rock CL, Doyle C, Demark-Wahnefried W, et al. Nutrition and physical activity guidelines for cancer survivors. CA Cancer J Clin. 2012;62:275–6.
14. Denlinger CS, Ligibel JA, Are M, Baker KS, Demark-Wahnefried W, Dizon D, et al. Survivorship: immunizations and prevention of infections, version 2.2014. J Natl Compr Cancer Netw. 2014;12(8):1098–111.
15. John GM, Hershman DL, Falci L, Shi Z, Tsai W-Y, Greenlee H. Complementary and alternative medicine use among US cancer survivors. J Cancer Surviv. 2016;10:850–64.
16. Armes J, Crowe M, Colbourne L, Morgan H, Murrells T, Oakley C, Palmer N, Ream E, Young A, Richardson A. Patients supportive care needs beyond the end of cancer treatment: a prospective, longitudinal survey. J Clin Oncol. 2009;27:6172–9.
17. Simard S, Thewes B, Humphris G, Dixon M, Hayden C, Mireskandari S, Ozakinci G. Fear of cancer recurrence in adult cancer survivors: a systematic review of quantitative studies. J Cancer Surviv. 2013;7:300–22.
18. Butow P, Sharpe L, Thewes B, Turner J, Gilchrist J, Beith J. Fear of cancer recurrence: a practical guide for clinicians. Oncology (Williston Park). 2018;32:32–8.
19. Yi JC, Syrjala KL. Anxiety and depression in cancer survivors. Med Clin N Am. 2017;101:1099–113.
20. Bower JE, Bak K, Berger A, et al. Screening, assessment, and management of fatigue in adult survivors of cancer: an American Society of Clinical Oncology Clinical Practice Guideline Adaptation. J Clin Oncol. 2014;32:1840–50.
21. Janelsins MC, Heckler CE, Peppone LJ, et al. Cognitive complaints in survivors of breast Cancer after chemotherapy compared with age-matched controls: an analysis from a nationwide, multicenter, prospective longitudinal study. J Clin Oncol. 2017;35:506–14.
22. Falk SJ, Dizon DS. Sexual dysfunction in women with cancer. Fertil Steril. 2013;100:916–21.
23. Morris L, Do V, Chard J, Brand A. Radiation-induced vaginal stenosis: current perspectives. Int J Women's Health. 2017;9:273–9.
24. Baumgart J, Nilsson K, Evers AS, Kallak TK, Poromaa IS. Sexual dysfunction in women on adjuvant endocrine therapy after breast cancer. Menopause. 2013;20:162–8.
25. Guy GP Jr, Ekwueme D, Yabroff K, Dowling E, Li C, Rodriguez J, Moor JD, Virgo K. The economic burden of cancer survivorship among adults in the United States. Value Health. 2013. https://doi.org/10.1016/j.jval.2013.03.666.
26. Bregendahl S, Emmertsen KJ, Lous J, Laurberg S. Bowel dysfunction after low anterior resection with and without neoadjuvant therapy for rectal cancer: a population-based cross-sectional study. Color Dis. 2013. https://doi.org/10.1111/codi.12244.
27. Emmertsen KJ, Laurberg S. Impact of bowel dysfunction on quality of life after sphincter-preserving resection for rectal cancer. Br J Surg. 2013;100:1377–87.
28. Krouse RS, Herrinton LJ, Grant M, et al. Health-related quality of life among long-term rectal cancer survivors with an ostomy: manifestations by sex. J Clin Oncol. 2009;27:4664–70.
29. Bekaii-Saab T, El-Rayes BF, Pawlik TM. Handbook of gastrointestinal cancers: evidence-based treatment and multidisciplinary patient care. New York: Springer Publishing Company; 2020.
30. Mols F, Beijers T, Vreugdenhil G, Poll-Franse LVD. Chemotherapy-induced peripheral neuropathy and its association with quality of life: a systematic review. Support Care Cancer. 2014;22:2261–9.
31. Gillespie LD, Robertson MC, Gillespie WJ, Sherrington C, Gates S, Clemson LM, Lamb SE. Interventions for preventing falls in older people living in the community. Cochrane Database Syst Rev. 2012. https://doi.org/10.1002/14651858.cd007146.pub3.
32. Hershman DL, Lacchetti C, Dworkin RH, et al. Prevention and management of chemotherapy-induced peripheral neuropathy in survivors of adult cancers: American Society of Clinical Oncology Clinical Practice Guideline. J Clin Oncol. 2014;32:1941–67.
33. Yusef SW, et al. Radiation-induced heart disease: a clinical update. Cardiol Res Pract. 2011;2011:317659.
34. Li K, Giustini D, Seely D. A systematic review of acupuncture for chemotherapy-induced peripheral neuropathy. Curr Oncol. 2019. https://doi.org/10.3747/co.26.4261.

35. Armenian SH, Lacchetti C, Lenihan D. Prevention and monitoring of cardiac dysfunction in survivors of adult cancers: American Society of Clinical Oncology Clinical Practice Guideline Summary. J Oncol Pract. 2017;13(4):270–5.
36. Burstein HJ, Lacchetti C, Anderson H, et al. Adjuvant endocrine therapy for women with hormone receptor–positive breast cancer: ASCO clinical practice guideline focused update. J Clin Oncol. 2019;37:423–38.
37. Henry NL, Unger JM, Schott AF, et al. Randomized, multicenter, placebo-controlled clinical trial of duloxetine versus placebo for aromatase inhibitor–associated arthralgias in early-stage breast cancer: SWOG S1202. J Clin Oncol. 2018;36:326–32.
38. Hadji P, Aapro MS, Body J-J, et al. Management of Aromatase Inhibitor-Associated Bone Loss (AIBL) in postmenopausal women with hormone sensitive breast cancer: joint position statement of the IOF, CABS, ECTS, IEG, ESCEO, IMS, and SIOG. J Bone Oncol. 2017;7:1–12.
39. Matthews A, Stanway S, Farmer RE, Strongman H, Thomas S, Lyon AR, Smeeth L, Bhaskaran K. Long term adjuvant endocrine therapy and risk of cardiovascular disease in female breast cancer survivors: systematic review. BMJ. 2018. https://doi.org/10.1136/bmj.k3845.
40. Practice Bulletin No. 126: management of gynecologic issues in women with breast cancer. Obstet Gynecol. 2012;119:666–82.
41. Donneyong MM, Bykov K, Bosco-Levy P, Dong Y-H, Levin R, Gagne JJ. Risk of mortality with concomitant use of tamoxifen and selective serotonin reuptake inhibitors: multi-database cohort study. BMJ. 2016;354:i5014.
42. Salloum RG, Hornbrook MC, Fishman PA, Ritzwoller DP, Rossetti MCO, Lafata JE. Adherence to surveillance care guidelines after breast and colorectal cancer treatment with curative intent. Cancer. 2012;118:5644–51.
43. Potosky AL, Han PKJ, Rowland J, Klabunde CN, Smith T, Aziz N, Earle C, Ayanian JZ, Ganz PA, Stefanek M. Differences between primary care physicians' and oncologists' knowledge, attitudes and practices regarding the care of cancer survivors. J Gen Intern Med. 2011;26:1403–10.
44. Yang EJ, Lim J-Y, Rah UW, Kim YB. Effect of a pelvic floor muscle training program on gynecologic cancer survivors with pelvic floor dysfunction: a randomized controlled trial. Gynecol Oncol. 2012;125:705–11.

# Obesity and Aging

Parvathi Perumareddi, Joanna Drowos, and Elizabeth Lownik

**Key Points**
- The prevalence of obesity in older women is increasing. Non-Hispanic Black women and women with lower education level are at particularly high risk.
- Waist circumference is a better predictor of obesity-associated risk than body mass index (BMI) in older women.
- Using nonjudgmental and inclusive language and motivational interviewing techniques will optimize productive discussions with patients about their weight.
- The goal of obesity treatment is to mitigate associated risks and improve function and quality of life.
- Weight loss may improve hypertension, hyperlipidemia, progression from impaired glucose tolerance to diabetes, urinary incontinence, sleep apnea, depression, physical functioning, quality of life, joint pain, and mobility.
- Older women are vulnerable to sarcopenia, osteoporosis, and nutritional deficiency when attempting weight loss. Gradual weight loss and maintaining adequate protein intake are important.

---

P. Perumareddi (✉)
Charles E Schmidt College of Medicine at Florida Atlantic University, Boca Raton, FL, USA
e-mail: pperumar@health.fau.edu

J. Drowos
Division of Family Medicine, Department of Integrated Medical Science, Charles E Schmidt College of Medicine at Florida Atlantic University, Boca Raton, FL, USA
e-mail: jdrowos@health.fau.edu

E. Lownik
Department of Family Medicine and Community Health, University of Wisconsin School of Medicine and Public Health and Dean Medical Group/SSM Health, Madison, WI, USA

- Lifestyle modifications including behavior changes, increased physical activity, and decreased caloric intake are first-line recommendations.
- Intensive lifestyle interventions to support patients in their weight loss are available in the community, commercially, and online.
- Additional treatment options include pharmacotherapy and bariatric surgery.
- Obesity is an important topic to address throughout the lifespan, with specific changes being recognized and tailored as a woman ages.

## Introduction

The obesity epidemic continues to grow in the United States and worldwide, across ethnicities and age groups. By 2030, it is estimated that almost half of US adults will be obese and almost one quarter will be severely obese [1]. In 2010, more than one-third of adults aged 65 and older were obese, and as the Baby Boomer generation ages, it is anticipated that the percentage of older people with obesity will also rise [2, 3].

The prevalence of obesity is higher in women than men and disproportionately affects non-Hispanic Black women and those with lower levels of educational attainment (Fig. 7.1) [3]. Approximately half of non-Hispanic Black women aged 65 and older are obese. Obesity is associated with multiple comorbidities and can reduce functionality and negatively impact quality of life.

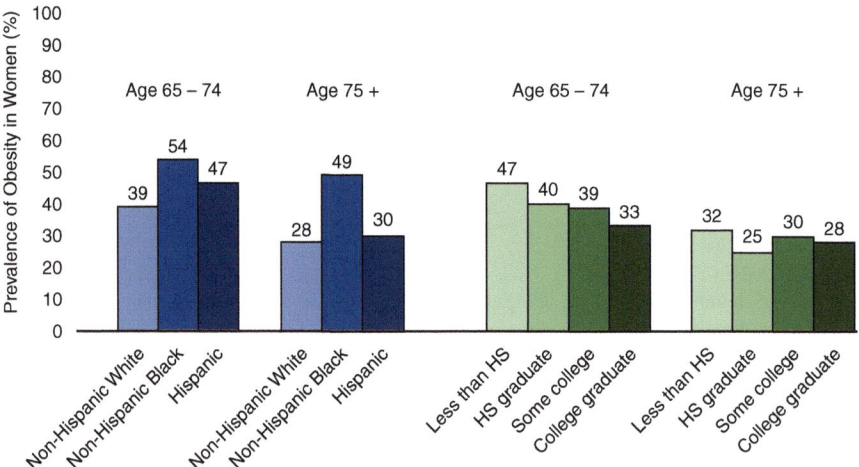

**Fig. 7.1** Prevalence of obesity among US adult women over 65 years old by age, race, and education, 2007–2010. This figure uses data from the National Center for Health Statistics as reported by Fakouri et al. in 2012 [3];. HS, high school

# 7 Obesity and Aging

> **Case**
> Beth S. is a 65-year-old woman whom you know well. She is following up for a new diagnosis of prediabetes (HgA1C of 6.1). She also has well-controlled hypertension, elevated lipids, and obesity (BMI 35). She tells you that she has tried diets in the past but none have worked. She wonders why it is so hard to lose weight.

## Pathophysiology of Obesity in Older Women

Body weight is influenced by a combination of genetics, metabolism, environment, behavior, and culture (Box 7.1) [4, 5].

Obesity results from the storage of excess energy as fat when caloric intake exceeds caloric requirements. As we become more sedentary with aging, our level of physical activity declines. As our basic metabolic rate decreases with age, our daily caloric need declines so that older adults need 300–500 fewer kCal/day than younger adults [6]. Importantly, despite this decrease in daily caloric consumption, older adults have unique nutritional requirements because of their vulnerability to diseases such as osteoporosis (See also Chapter 3) and sarcopenia. Box 7.2 describes the obesity paradox, whereby a higher weight in older adults may actually benefit health where it would worsen health in younger adults.

Sarcopenia, the progressive loss of skeletal mass with increasing age, can predispose older adults to sarcopenic obesity. Illness or inactivity can lead to loss of muscle mass, while body fat is preserved and redistributed. Sarcopenic obesity is associated with functional decline, frailty, and higher morbidity and mortality. It is thus recommended that older adults maintain or even increase their daily protein consumption.

> **Box 7.1 How Do Genetics, Environmental, and Behavioral Factors Contribute to Obesity?**
> - Genome-wide association studies have identified more than 140 genetic chromosomal regions related to obesity. Only a few of these genes have a large effect on BMI (such as genes encoding leptin and melanocortin signaling). It is thus likely that familial trends in obesity represent both genetic and environmental influences.
> - Humans in environments with high food availability and reminders of food through conditioned stimuli and media cues may struggle with overeating.
> - Altered connectivity between the salience and inhibitory network and other cortical areas (hedonic control) as well as interactions with the hypothalamus (homeostatic controls) can interfere with processing emotional control and reward-based decision making in food choices.

> **Box 7.2 What Is the Obesity Paradox?** [10]
> - Obesity in younger adults shortens life expectancy, but in older adults, the optimal weight for survival increases with age.
> - Above age 75, the relative risk of all-cause mortality decreases with increasing BMI, resulting in a U-shaped curve where risk of death increases at both extremes of BMI (too low and too high).
> - The effects of weight loss in older adults remain controversial with an emphasis on physical function showing benefit rather than absolute weight loss.

Hormonal changes, such as reduced production of growth hormone and testosterone, and decreased responsiveness to thyroid hormone and leptin, predispose older adults to obesity. For older women, these changes may be more pronounced. Women have more body fat as a percentage of body weight than men do from puberty onward and gain more fat during adult life than men. Pregnancy may result in modest but adverse changes in body weight and fat distribution that persist throughout the lifespan [7, 8]. Following menopause, reduced estrogen states further decrease the lipolytic effects of an energy negative state [6].

Common medications can contribute to weight gain in older adults, including many that treat common comorbidities such as diabetes, depression, and hypertension. The Obesity Action Coalition has a helpful resource that includes a table of drugs that may be associated with weight gain and suggested alternatives that may have a more favorable impact on weight. While underlying diseases such as hypothyroidism, polycystic ovarian syndrome, Cushing's syndrome, and Prader–Willi syndrome can lead to obesity, these causes are less common in older adults.

Obesity is associated with numerous physiologic changes that impact overall health [9]. Secretion of excess adipokines from white adipose tissue results in insulin resistance, diabetes mellitus, dyslipidemia, hypertension, and atherosclerosis. Obesity affects inflammation and is thus a risk factor for breast, colon, endometrial, esophageal, hepatocellular, and renal cancer. Obesity enhances degenerative joint disease not only from increased weight bearing on joints, but also from the damaging effect of inflammatory adipokines such as resistin on joint synovia and muscle function. Extra adipose tissue in the upper respiratory tract and hypopharynx predisposes to sleep apnea, impaired ventilation, secondary hypoxia, and hypercapnia. Finally, obesity negatively affects functional ability, resulting in social isolation and decreased ability to perform activities of daily living. Obesity is associated with incontinence and depression, and associated stigma can lead to worsening social isolation.

## Clinical Risks of Obesity

Obesity increases the risk of cardiovascular disease, sleep apnea, nonalcoholic fatty liver disease, osteoarthritis, depression, urinary incontinence, and impaired quality of life in older women.

Women with obesity have a higher mortality risk if they also have coronary heart disease, type 2 diabetes mellitus (T2DM), or sleep apnea.

It is important to identify modifiable risk factors for cardiovascular disease in women with obesity that can independently reduce their risk of death. These factors are as follows:

- Hypertension
- Hyperlipidemia
- Impaired glucose tolerance
- Sleep apnea
- Tobacco use

*Importantly, weight loss may improve hypertension, hyperlipidemia, progression from impaired glucose tolerance to diabetes, urinary incontinence, sleep apnea, depression, physical functioning, quality of life, joint pain, and mobility.*

## Diagnosing and Evaluating Persons with Obesity

It is important to discuss obesity using sensitive and inclusive language. It is useful to frame the discussion around managing chronic medical conditions like diabetes and hypertension. In a survey of 390 patients with obesity with a mean age of 51 years old, the term "weight" was preferred over the "obesity," "heavy," and "fat," which were perceived to as judgmental; "BMI" was also considered an acceptable term [11].

Most patients have been through the process over many years of losing (and gaining back) weight, so we should understand that the issue is almost never lack of insight. Often times, the bigger challenge is maintaining (not achieving) a healthy weight. Many patients are already frustrated and impatient with themselves and their lack of sustained progress and it is vital to impart understanding, respect, and empathy in the discussion about their weight.

Motivational interviewing can be a helpful technique when broaching the topic of weight. Motivational interviewing has four key components: (1) expressing empathy and not arguing; (2) developing discrepancy; (3) rolling with (not fighting) resistance; and (4) supporting self-efficacy. In this process, the provider assesses the patient's readiness for and interest in making lifestyle changes and guides discussion and action based on her current state of mind and stage of contemplation [12].

Best practices for building trust and improving conversations around weight include the following:

- Share the agenda. "Is it OK if we talk about ways to improve your health and quality of life?"
- Raise the issue. "I would like to talk about your weight."
- Be respectful and express empathy.
- Build on what you hear (ask, tell, ask). "What have you tried in the past? It sounds like losing weight has been important to you for a long time. You've tried very hard and have been frustrated and disappointed. Can you tell me about some moments that were rewarding?"
- Cultivate change talk. "It sounds like you are ready to make a change."
- Guide toward a specific plan. "How would you feel about a referral to a program to support you in making these changes? There are in-person and online programs, and they have helped a lot of my patients."

Training in motivational interviewing is helpful not only for supporting patients in behavior change around weight, but also for smoking cessation, mental health, substance use disorders, and diabetes. The Obesity Medicine Academy offers a webinar for healthcare providers with limited experience using motivational interviewing. Trusted resources about motivational interviewing can be found here.

## Classifying Obesity in Older Women

Body mass index (BMI), measured in kilograms per meter squared, does not take into account body composition, making it less accurate in older persons, whose fat-free mass (FFM) is lower than that of younger adults [13]. As muscle mass declines, BMI can underestimate obesity. Older women may also lose height from vertebral compression fractures, further complicating the interpretation of BMI in this population.

When using BMI to define obesity (Fig. 7.2), a BMI of 30 kg/m$^2$ or more is obese. Obesity is subdivided into classes, with BMI of 30–34.9 kg/m$^2$ being Class 1, 35–39.9 kg/m$^2$ Class 2, and BMI ≥40 kg/m$^2$ Class 3, also known as severe, extreme, or massive obesity.

Waist circumference correlates highly with total fat and intra-abdominal fat and is a better predictor of obesity-related risk in women. Waist circumference should be measured in women with a BMI between 25 and 35 kg/m$^2$. A waist

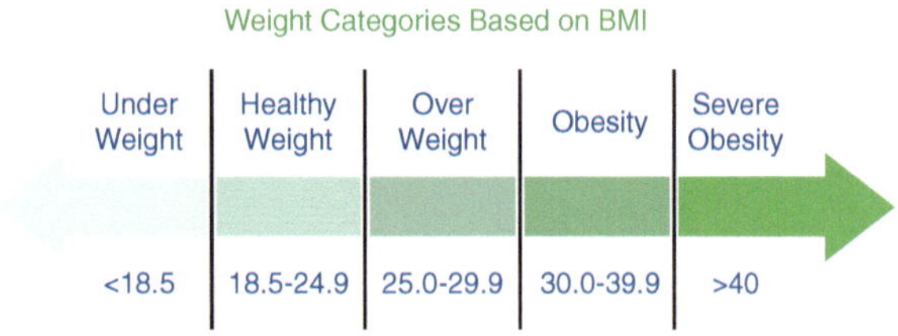

**Fig. 7.2** Weight categories based on BMI

Weight Categories Based on BMI

| Under Weight | Healthy Weight | Over Weight | Obesity | Severe Obesity |
|---|---|---|---|---|
| <18.5 | 18.5-24.9 | 25.0-29.9 | 30.0-39.9 | >40 |

circumference of >35″ (88 cm) correlates with increased cardiometabolic risk. Of note, Asian women are at increased risk with a BMI > 23 kg/m$^2$ and a waist circumference >31 in (80 cm).

Obesity-related comorbidities should be assessed and treated in any woman with a BMI ≥ 25 kg/m$^2$.

A waist circumference should be measured and a weight and lifestyle history obtained. If a patient is not ready to make lifestyle changes to achieve weight loss, she should be advised to avoid weight gain, and her weight, BMI, and waist circumference should be measured at least annually.

Table 7.1 outlines the diagnostic evaluation of women with obesity. The minimum basic evaluation of a woman with obesity includes history and physical, including careful medication review, fasting glucose or Hemoglobin A1c, thyroid stimulating hormone, liver enzymes (ALT, AST), and fasting lipid panel (total cholesterol, LDL, HDL, and triglycerides) so that you can further characterize her risk and guide her treatment.

All patients with overweight and obesity should be clinically evaluated for complications and comorbidities such as cardiovascular disease, diabetes mellitus,

**Table 7.1** Diagnostic evaluation of women with obesity [14]

| Complications of obesity | Recommended evaluation |
|---|---|
| *Metabolic syndrome* | Waist circumference (https://www.youtube.com/watch?v=3XNBeam5NoM) |
| *Hypertension* | Blood pressure (https://www.youtube.com/watch?v=-LqKmrmaHsk) |
| *Diabetes mellitus type 2* | Fasting serum glucose/hemoglobin A1C |
| *Hyperlipidemia* | Lipid panel (total cholesterol, triglycerides, high-density lipoprotein (HDL), and low-density lipoprotein (LDL)) |
| *Non-alcoholic fatty liver disease* | Liver function (total protein, albumin, bilirubin (total and direct), alkaline phosphatase (ALP), aspartate aminotransferase (AST), alanine aminotransferase (ALT)) |
| *Obstructive sleep apnea* | STOP BANG, sleep study (See also Chapter 8) (http://www.stopbang.ca/osa/screening.php) |
| *Urinary incontinence* | Symptom assessment (i.e., questionnaire for female urinary incontinence diagnosis (QUID) (See also Chapter 11): https://www.ncbi.nlm.nih.gov/pmc/articles/PMC2891326/ |
| *Degenerative joint disease* | Symptom assessment (i.e., arthritis symptom checker: https://arthritis.ca/about-arthritis/signs-of-arthritis/symptom-checker/) |
| *Depression* | PHQ-9 (https://hign.org/consultgeri/try-this-series/geriatric-depression-scale-gds), Geriatric Depression Scale (https://hign.org/consultgeri/try-this-series/geriatric-depression-scale-gds) (See also Chapter 4.) |
| *Binge eating disorder* | Binge eating disorder screener (BEDS-7: https://www.vyvansepro.com/documents/Adult-Binge-Eating-Disorder-Patient-Screener.pdf) |

nonalcoholic fatty liver disease, obstructive sleep apnea, and depression (see Table 7.1). Appropriate follow-up and treatment for identified comorbidities should be pursued as medically indicated. Underlying contributing conditions such as hypothyroidism should be explored where indicated, and a thorough history including recent health changes, reduction in functional status, or social factors that may be contributing to weight gain should be obtained.

## Medication Reconciliation

Medications may cause weight gain via various mechanisms:

- Fluid retention
- Stimulation of appetite
- Lowering of metabolism
- Stimulation of fat storage
- Impaired exercise tolerance

Given the importance of reducing polypharmacy in older adults, a risk-benefit assessment of each medicine is of inherent value, and can also reduce the risk of medication-related weight gain. Sometimes, medications associated with weight gain can be substituted for weight-neutral options; occasionally, a lower dose of a particular medication can attenuate weight gain. Box 7.3 provides a list of medications that may have an impact on weight.

Prior to undergoing a weight loss program, postmenopausal women should have their baseline bone mineral density tested. Intervention should begin with a weight history, previous strategies for weight loss, amount of physical activity and functional barriers, sleep, and social support. Older adults are particularly vulnerable to food

---

**Box 7.3 Medications That May Impact Weight**
- Diabetes therapies (insulin, sulfonylureas, and thiazolidinediones)
- Selective Serotonin Reuptake Inhibitors (SSRIS)
- Anticonvulsants (including gabapentin)
- Oral corticosteroids
- Hormone therapy (estrogen and progesterone)
- Tricyclic antidepressants
- Antihistamines
- Beta-blockers
- Antipsychotics
- Lithium

# 7 Obesity and Aging

insecurity and social isolation and should be screened and appropriately addressed if identified [6]. Cognitive impairment or reduced executive functioning is also important to identify and to modify patient goals and clinician approach accordingly.

> **Case (Continued)**
> Beth wants to talk to you today about losing weight so that she doesn't have to start on medications for diabetes. She does not do much exercise, but recently got a pedometer. She takes 3500 steps per day on average. You jointly talk about having her do a daily food log, schedule her for an appointment with the nutritionist, and set a goal for her to increase her daily steps by 1000 every week. She feels like it will be challenging to make these changes on her own.

## Intensive Lifestyle Interventions for Weight Loss

According to the Guidelines for the Management of Overweight and Obesity in Adults [15], the first-line treatment for patients who are ready to make lifestyle changes to achieve weight loss is an intensive lifestyle intervention for a minimum of 6 months. An intensive lifestyle intervention (Fig. 7.3) includes (1) a reduced-calorie diet, (2) increased physical activity, and (3) behavior therapy [16].

Such intensive lifestyle interventions may be offered within a medical setting by staff such as registered dietitians but are rarely performed by a primary care provider because of their intensity. These in-person interventions typically result in a weight loss of approximately 8 kg or 8% of initial weight and improve health and quality of life; programs delivered by telephone, internet, or smartphone are also effective but usually result in less weight loss [16]. If your health system does not offer an intensive lifestyle intervention, you can refer patients to community-based programs, commercial programs, or weight management apps (see Fig. 7.3). The most extensively tested and proven one of these interventions is the Diabetes Prevention Program (DPP), disseminated by the Centers for Disease Control and Prevention (CDC) and the YMCA. To be eligible for the DPP, patients must have evidence of prediabetes without an existing or prior diagnosis of DM (Box 7.4).

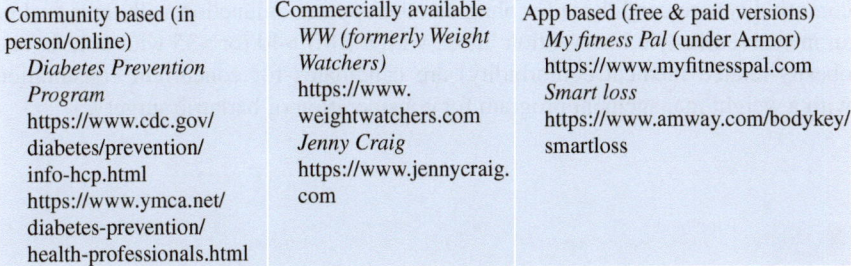

| Community based (in person/online) | Commercially available | App based (free & paid versions) |
|---|---|---|
| Diabetes Prevention Program https://www.cdc.gov/diabetes/prevention/info-hcp.html https://www.ymca.net/diabetes-prevention/health-professionals.html | WW (formerly Weight Watchers) https://www.weightwatchers.com Jenny Craig https://www.jennycraig.com | My fitness Pal (under Armor) https://www.myfitnesspal.com Smart loss https://www.amway.com/bodykey/smartloss |

**Fig. 7.3** Intensive lifestyle interventions for weight loss

> **Box 7.4 Diabetes Prevention Program Eligibility**
> - ≥18 years old with BMI ≥25 (≥23 if Asian)
> - No prior diagnosis of DM
> - Evidence of prediabetes (any one of these qualifies)*
>   - Hgb A1c 5.7–6.4% within last year
>   - Fasting BG 100–125 mg/dL in last year
>   - 75 g GTT → 140–199 mg/dL (2 h) in last year
>   - History of gestational DM
>   - High risk for type 2 DM on Prediabetes Risk Test
>
> * Medicare beneficiaries must have blood test clinically administered in last year to qualify (self-reporting not allowed)

> **Box 7.5 Intensive Behavior Therapy for Obesity**
> Medicare pays for this!
> Intensive Behavior Therapy (IBT) for Obesity
> For Medicare patients with a BMI > 30 kg/m$^2$, face-to-face counseling for obesity (15 min) can be billed under the code G0447 in a primary care setting for:
> - One visit every week for 4 weeks.
> - One visit every other week for months 2–6.
> - One visit every month for months 7–12 if the patient has lost at least 3 kg (6.6 lb) during the first 6 months.

Primary care providers can also provide and be reimbursed for intensive behavioral therapy (Box 7.5) that includes a dietary assessment and counseling to promote high intensity changes related to nutrition and exercise, either in conjunction with a formal intensive lifestyle intervention or independently if this is not available locally.

Those patients with a BMI >30 (or >27 with at least one obesity-related medical comorbidity) are candidates for pharmacotherapy in conjunction with their trial of an intensive lifestyle intervention; those with a BMI >40 (or >35 with at least one obesity-related medical comorbidity) are candidates for concurrent consultation with a weight management program for consideration of bariatric surgery.

> **Case (Continued)**
> Beth opts for referral to a Diabetes Prevention Program near you. While she is a candidate for pharmacotherapy or referral to a bariatric surgeon based on her BMI and medical comorbidities, she is motivated to avoid additional medication and declines consult with bariatric surgery right now. You schedule a follow-up appointment for her in 3 months to monitor her progress. At that visit, she is very proud of her progress and asks whether the same program would be appropriate for her mother, who is 92.

## Treating Obesity in the Much Older Adult

In the elderly, because weight loss can actually worsen comorbidities, it is important to assess whether and to what extent an individual patient may benefit from weight loss. Improved health depends not only on weight loss but also on correlation with functionality. Though data are limited, a combination of lifestyle modifications is likely the best approach to weight loss for much older women. *The goal is to create a calorie deficit of 300–500 kCal /day through a combination of dietary changes and exercise.*

A combination of aerobic activity, resistance training, and weight management (through dietary calorie reduction) has been shown to improve weight loss, frailty, cardiovascular fitness, and functional ability in adults over 65 with a BMI >30 [17].

## Physical Activity

The American College of Sports Medicine suggests at least 150 min of low-to-moderate intensity aerobic activity in all people, including older adults. Those with reduced cardiovascular fitness or other physical limitations should be advised to break up the 150 minutes into small, attainable increments and build from there as they are able. It is important to incorporate both aerobic exercise, preferably weight bearing to aid in bone health/density, and resistance training, which benefit muscle strength, bone density, and functional capacity for everyday movement and activity, which is helpful to prevent falls.

The National Institute on Aging has a free exercise guide to download for patients to use at home: https://www.nia.nih.gov/health/publication/exercise-physical-activity/introduction

## Dietary Changes

While calorie reduction relative to calorie consumption results in weight loss, losing lean muscle mass is a concern for the elderly. Ensuring adequate nutrition helps preserve muscle mass in this vulnerable population, so weight loss at a measured pace is more desirable than rapid weight loss. Patients should be advised to track calories by hand or using an app (see Fig. 7.3 on Intensive Lifestyle Interventions above).

Dietary protein is particularly important for older adults and contributes to muscle mass, reserve capacity, skin resilience, immune function, and healing [18, 19]. In fact, observational data show a correlation between higher protein intake and better physical function and muscle strength in older women [20].

While attempting weight loss, older women should get at least the recommended daily amount (RDA) of protein, if not more, to maintain muscle mass [21]. The RDA for this age group is 0.8–1.2 g protein/kg body weight per day. Some experts suggest that the RDA for older adults should be >1.2 g per kg/day, especially given that a high protein diet has not been shown to have a negative impact on renal and bone health in humans [22].

Timing of dietary protein intake is also likely important, and older women should be advised to consume protein-rich foods with each meal to maximize muscle protein synthesis and combat sarcopenic changes [23]. Dietary animal protein contains valuable iron, vitamin B-12, folic acid, biotin, and eggs that are particularly nutritious and affordable [19].

It is best to coordinate with a clinical nutritionist or a registered dietitian when recommending weight loss in older adults so that they can help patients consider their ideal daily calorie deficit, provide recommendations about adequate protein intake and low glycemic foods, and educate patients about how to read and interpret nutritional labels, in particular looking at serving sizes and macronutrients (percentages of proteins, fats, and carbohydrates).

> **Case (Continued)**
> At her 6-month follow-up visit, Beth's weight loss has plateaued, though her HgA1C has gone down to 5.8. She is now getting, on an average, 7000 steps a day and feels better. She is ready to talk about other options. She is hesitant to start on medications due to potential side effects, but agrees to go to see the weight management program to discuss a medically supervised very low calorie diet.

## Next Steps and Other Treatments

If a patient achieves at least 5% weight reduction after 6 months of an intensive lifestyle intervention, she should then be transitioned at weight loss maintenance program including at least monthly counseling with a trained interventionist for at least 1 year [16]. While patients may consider their obesity a temporary problem, it is important to discuss obesity as a chronic medical condition and emphasize the importance of long-term adherence to treatment.

If a patient does not achieve at least 5% weight loss after 6 months of an intensive lifestyle intervention, she is a candidate for pharmacotherapy or referral for consultation with a weight management program for consideration of bariatric surgery, usually in that order. While we need more data about pharmacotherapy and bariatric surgery in older adults, older age should not preclude these advanced options for appropriately selected patients [24]. Once goal weight loss is achieved, patients should be transitioned to a weight loss maintenance program as described above.

## Medications for Treatment of Obesity

There are five medications that are currently available and FDA approved for weight loss (see Table 7.2).[1] Though there is insufficient evidence to definitively recommend these medications in older adults [14], preliminary data and the known pharmacologic profiles of the medications suggest that there is minimal difference between older and younger populations [6]. That said, the risk of polypharmacy in older patients should not be underestimated, and a new medication should not be prescribed lightly.

In conjunction with lifestyle change, medication for weight loss can be considered for all patients with a BMI $\geq$ 30 kg/m$^2$, or with a BMI of $\geq$27 kg/m$^2$, and at least one associated comorbid medical condition such as hypertension, dyslipidemia, type 2 diabetes mellitus (T2DM), and obstructive sleep apnea [25].

Overall evidence of efficacy of weight loss medication is modest but significant, with effects averaging 5–9% of body weight loss when prescribed along with adherence to lifestyle changes [25]. In general, the FDA approved antiobesity medications that can be considered for any adult for whom diet and lifestyle changes are inadequate. The risk of side effects should always be considered; however, medication should be used with caution and close monitoring. Efficacy and safety of medications should be assessed after the first 3 months. The medication is considered successful if a patient has lost >5% of their body weight by that time [25]. If this has not occurred, stop the medication.

Insurance must also be taken into consideration, as coverage for antiobesity medication is poor. In 2017, a study that analyzed commercial healthcare plan coverage of antiobesity medications found that only 11% included some kind of coverage [26], and at the time of publication there is no Medicare coverage.

---

[1] A sixth medication, Lorcaserin, was FDA approved for treatment of obesity in 2012 but was taken off the market in February 2020 because of associated increased risk of cancer.

**Table 7.2** FDA-approved pharmacotherapy for obesity

| Drug | Dosage | Mechanism of action | Side effects | Contraindications |
|---|---|---|---|---|
| Phentermine* | 30–37.5 mg/d | Norepinephrine-releasing agent | Dry mouth, constipation, anxiety, tachycardia, hypertension, insomnia, dysphoria, tremor, and psychosis | Glaucoma, heart disease, hyperthyroidism, and arrhythmias |
| Phentermine/Topiramate (ER) | 3.75 mg/23 mg ER/d (starting) 7.5 mg /46 mg ER/d (recommended) 15 mg/92 mg ER/d (high dose) | Norepinephrine-releasing agent/ GABA receptor modulation | See above, also paresthesia, mental cloudiness, and fatigue | See above |
| Orlistat | 60–120 mg TID | Pancreatic and gastric lipase inhibitor | Decreased absorption of fat-soluble vitamins, steatorrhea, oily spotting, flatulence, and fecal incontinence | Cholestasis and malabsorption syndrome |
| Bupropion/Naltrexone | 32 mg/360 mg two tablets QID (titrate up) | Reuptake inhibitor of dopamine and norepinephrine (bupropion) and opioid antagonist (naltrexone) | CNS effects, nausea, vomiting, constipation, headache, and dizziness | Seizure disorder, severe hepatic impairment, and concurrent chronic opioid prescription |
| Liraglutide | 3.0 mg injectable | GLP-1 agonist | Nausea, vomiting, diarrhea, and hypoglycemia | History of medullary thyroid cancer or multiple endocrine neoplasia type 2 |

*Phentermine alone is only FDA approved for use for 3 months

In spite of the lack of insurance coverage, cost, and side effects of antiobesity medication, clinicians can benefit their patients by thinking of potential synergy for other clinical applications. GLP-1 agonists, such as liraglutide, have shown significant benefit for diabetes control, and also have the benefit of weight loss. Similarly, a patient with depression and/or chronic pain may benefit from a combination of buprenorphine and naltrexone.

## Surgery

Bariatric surgery is an effective and well-validated treatment for obesity and related comorbidities in the general population. The majority of studies evaluating the efficacy and safety of bariatric surgery have excluded patients aged >60. Given the known increased perioperative risk with age, conflict exists regarding the role of surgery in this population [24]. However, a meta-analysis including over 8000 patients aged 60 years or older who underwent Roux-en-Y gastric bypass or sleeve gastrectomy determined that outcomes and complication rates of bariatric surgery in this population are comparable to patients aged <60, with pooled mean excess weight loss of 53.7% and diabetes resolution 54.5% at 1 year [27]. The decision to refer a woman for consideration of bariatric surgery should be individualized based on her overall health status, goals, and personal preferences, regardless of age.

Patients who are interested and appropriate candidates should be counseled that bariatric surgery may not be as effective for weight loss and remission of diabetes or hypertension for patients >60 years of age as it is for younger patients [28]. Insurance coverage should be confirmed (Box 7.6) and chronic disease control should be optimized to the extent possible, along with the screening for undiagnosed mental health disorder, nutritional deficiency, and cognitive impairment, prior to surgery. Adequate social support is essential in the immediate postoperative period. Dietary protein and weight bearing physical activity is important in the postoperative period to reduce the risk of sarcopenia.

> **Box 7.6 Bariatric Surgery Requirements for Coverage by Medicare**
> - BMI $\geq 35$ kg/m$^2$ plus at least one obesity-related medical condition (diabetes, hypertension, coronary artery disease, sleep apnea, cardiomyopathy)
> - Trial and failure of other treatments

## Conclusion

The management of older women with obesity is complex, primarily due to risks of sarcopenia, osteoporosis, and nutritional deficiency in the setting of attempted weight loss. The goals of obesity treatment in older women include reducing the risk of associated chronic conditions and improving functionality and quality of life. Approach and management should be tailored to an individual patient and her specific comorbidities. A balanced approach of lifestyle modifications addressing behavior, diet, and exercise is a good starting point. Intensive lifestyle interventions are available in the community, commercially, and online. Additional treatment options include pharmacotherapy and bariatric surgery. Obesity is a chronic condition and an extremely important topic to address throughout the lifespan, with specific changes being recognized and tailored as a woman ages.

## References

1. Ward ZJ, Bleich SN, Cradock AL, Barrett JL, Giles CM, Flax C, et al. Projected U.S. state-level prevalence of adult obesity and severe obesity. N Engl J Med. 2019;381(25):2440–50.
2. McKee A, Morley JE. Obesity in the elderly. South Dartmouth: MDText. com, Inc; 2000.
3. Fakhouri TH, Ogden CL, Carroll MD, Kit BK, Flegal KM. Prevalence of obesity among older adults in the United States, 2007-2010. NCHS Data Brief 2012;(106):1–8.
4. Heymsfield SB, Wadden TA. Mechanisms, pathophysiology, and management of obesity. N Engl J Med. 2017;376(15):1492.
5. Cetin DC, Nasr G. Obesity in the elderly: more complicated than you think. Cleve Clin J Med. 2014;81(1):51–61.
6. Batsis JA, Zagaria AB. Addressing obesity in aging patients. Med Clin North Am. 2018;102(1):65–85.
7. Gunderson EP, Sternfeld B, Wellons MF, Whitmer RA, Chiang V, Quesenberry CP Jr, et al. Childbearing may increase visceral adipose tissue independent of overall increase in body fat. Obesity (Silver Spring). 2008;16(5):1078–84.
8. Mannan M, Doi SA, Mamun AA. Association between weight gain during pregnancy and postpartum weight retention and obesity: a bias-adjusted meta-analysis. Nutr Rev. 2013 Jun;71(6):343–52.
9. Redinger RN. The pathophysiology of obesity and its clinical manifestations. Gastroenterol Hepatol (N Y). 2007;3(11):856–63.
10. Gadde KM, Martin CK, Berthoud HR, Heymsfield SB. Obesity: pathophysiology and management. J Am Coll Cardiol. 2018;71(1):69–84.
11. Volger S, Vetter ML, Dougherty M, Panigrahi E, Egner R, Webb V, et al. Patients' preferred terms for describing their excess weight: discussing obesity in clinical practice. Obesity (Silver Spring). 2012;20(1):147–50.
12. Reims K, Ernst D. Using motivational interviewing to promote healthy weight. Fam Pract Manag. 2016;23(5):32–8.
13. Amarya S, Singh K, Sabharwal M. Health consequences of obesity in the elderly. J Clin Gerontol Geriatr. 2014;5(3):63–7.
14. Garvey WT, Mechanick JI, Brett EM, Garber AJ, Hurley DL, Jastreboff AM, et al. American Association of Clinical Endocrinologists and American College of Endocrinology comprehensive clinical practice guidelines for medical care of patients with obesity. Endocr Pract. 2016;22 Suppl 3:1–203.
15. Jensen MD, Ryan DH, Apovian CM, Ard JD, Comuzzie AG, Hu FB, et al. Managing overweight and obesity in adults: systematic evidence review from the obesity expert panel, 2013: National Heart, Lung and Blood Institute; 2013.
16. Webb VL, Wadden TA. Intensive lifestyle intervention for obesity: principles, practices, and results. Gastroenterology. 2017;152(7):1752–64.
17. Villareal DT, Aguirre L, Gurney AB, Waters DL, Sinacore DR, Colombo E, et al. Aerobic or resistance exercise, or both, in dieting obese older adults. N Engl J Med. 2017;376(20):1943–55.
18. Chernoff R. Dietary management for older subjects with obesity. Clin Geriatr Med. 2005;21(4):725–33, vi.
19. Chernoff R. Protein and older adults. J Am Coll Nutr. 2004;23(6 Suppl):627S–30S.
20. Isanejad M, Mursu J, Sirola J, Kroger H, Rikkonen T, Tuppurainen M, et al. Dietary protein intake is associated with better physical function and muscle strength among elderly women. Br J Nutr. 2016;115(7):1281–91.
21. Bales CW, Porter Starr KN. Obesity interventions for older adults: diet as a determinant of physical function. Adv Nutr. 2018;9(2):151–9.
22. Traylor DA, Gorissen SHM, Phillips SM. Perspective: protein requirements and optimal intakes in aging: are we ready to recommend more than the recommended daily allowance? Adv Nutr. 2018;9(3):171–82.

23. Deer RR, Volpi E. Protein intake and muscle function in older adults. Curr Opin Clin Nutr Metab Care. 2015;18(3):248–53.
24. Haywood C, Sumithran P. Treatment of obesity in older persons-a systematic review. Obes Rev. 2019;20(4):588–98.
25. Apovian CM, Aronne LJ, Bessesen DH, McDonnell ME, Murad MH, Pagotto U, et al. Pharmacological management of obesity: an endocrine society clinical practice guideline. J Clin Endocrinol Metab. 2015;100(2):342–62.
26. Gomez G, Stanford FC. US health policy and prescription drug coverage of FDA-approved medications for the treatment of obesity. Int J Obes. 2015;42(3):495–500.
27. Giordano S, Victorzon M. Bariatric surgery in elderly patients: a systematic review. Clin Interv Aging. 2015;10:1627–35.
28. Faucher P, Aron-Wisnewsky J, Ciangura C, Genser L, Torcivia A, Bouillot JL, et al. Changes in body composition, comorbidities, and nutritional status associated with lower weight loss after bariatric surgery in older subjects. Obes Surg. 2019;29(11):3589–95.

# Insomnia and Sleep Disorders in Older Women

## 8

Krishna M. Desai, Heather L. Paladine, and Nataliya Pilipenko

> **Key Points**
> - Sleep disorders can adversely affect a woman's quality of life and important areas of functioning.
> - Older women face unique underlying factors that contribute to poor sleep such as menopausal symptoms, lower urinary tract symptoms, chronic medical conditions, mood disorders, and dementia.
> - Women, especially older women, are at higher risk of insomnia and sleep disorders than men.
> - Cognitive behavioral therapy for insomnia (CBT-I) is the first-line therapy option for patients with insomnia.
> - Combining multiple nonpharmacotherapy treatments and medications is an effective strategy to manage sleep problems.

## Epidemiology, Causes, and Terminology

> **Case**
> Martha is a 59 year old who has been unable to get a restful night of sleep for 2 years. She has cut out her daily coffee and sleeps in a cool room, but still has trouble falling asleep and wakes up twice overnight. You take a detailed history.

K. M. Desai (✉) · H. L. Paladine · N. Pilipenko
Center for Family and Community Medicine,
Columbia University Irving Medical Center, New York, NY, USA
e-mail: kmd2180@cumc.columbia.edu; np2615@cumc.columbia.edu

## Epidemiology

Sleep problems are common, occurring in 25% of adults [1]. Women and older people, such as Martha, are more likely to have difficulty with sleep. Women are more commonly affected due to hormonal changes such as pregnancy and menopause, and because of a higher prevalence of depression and anxiety. There is also an increased risk of certain medical and psychiatric conditions that can make women more susceptible to sleep problems.

Insomnia is associated with a higher cardiovascular risk and higher prevalence of mental health problems. Sleep problems result in a lower quality of life, increased risk for suicide, increased risk for accidents and substance use, and decreased work performance [1].

## Definitions and Causes of Insomnia and Sleep Disorders

Box 8.1 lists the Diagnostic and Statistical Manual of Mental Disorders, 5th Edition (DSM-5) criteria for insomnia disorder [2]. Insomnia may increase the risk of medical conditions and vice versa [3].

> **Box 8.1 DSM-5 Criteria for Insomnia Disorder**
> - A predominant complaint of dissatisfaction with sleep quantity or quality, associated with one or more of the following symptoms:
>   - Difficulty initiating sleep.
>   - Difficulty maintaining sleep, characterized by frequent awakenings or problems returning to sleep after awakenings.
>   - Early morning awakening with inability to return to sleep.
> - The sleep disturbance causes clinically significant distress or impairment in social, occupational, educational, academic, behavioral, or other important areas of functioning.
> - The sleep difficulty occurs at least three nights per week.
> - The sleep difficulty is present for at least 3 months.
> - The sleep difficulty occurs despite adequate opportunity for sleep.
> - The insomnia is not better explained by and does not occur exclusively during the course of another sleep–wake disorder.
> - The insomnia is not attributable to the physiological effects of a substance.
> - Coexisting mental disorders and medical conditions do not adequately explain the predominant complaint of insomnia.

Box 8.2 lists common medical conditions that are associated with insomnia. These potential causes should be evaluated before considering treatment for insomnia.

Other underlying sleep disorders that patients may present with include hypersomnolence disorder, narcolepsy, breathing-related sleep disorders (obstructive sleep apnea or hypopnea, central sleep apnea, sleep-related hypoventilation), circadian rhythm sleep–wake disorders, and parasomnias (nonrapid eye movement sleep arousal disorders, nightmare disorder, rapid eye movement sleep behavior disorder, restless legs syndrome).

### Box 8.2 Conditions That May Contribute to Insomnia

| | |
|---|---|
| Medical conditions | Menopause symptoms such as hot flashes<br>Hyperthyroidism<br>Pain syndromes<br>Osteoarthritis<br>Gastroesophageal reflux disease (GERD)<br>Sleep apnea<br>Cardiopulmonary disease causing shortness of breath<br>Alzheimer's disease<br>Parkinson disease<br>Nocturia |
| Psychiatric conditions | Anxiety<br>Depression<br>Persistent complex bereavement disorder (grief)<br>Post-traumatic stress disorder (PTSD)<br>Psychosocial stressors |
| Medications | Stimulants, such as amphetamines and decongestants<br>Theophylline<br>Beta blockers<br>Levothyroxine<br>Some antidepressants, such as fluoxetine<br>Steroids |
| Other substances | Caffeine<br>Alcohol<br>Nicotine<br>Cocaine |

## Terminology

Commonly used terms related to sleep disorders are listed in Box 8.3. These definitions will help to evaluate and then treat Martha's sleep problems.

## Evaluation

> **Case (Continued)**
> Martha tells you that she has been having hot flashes that wake her up at nighttime. She often drinks two glasses of wine with dinner, and says that helps her sleep.

A person who presents with difficulty sleeping should have a detailed history including medical and psychiatric concerns. The history should include medical conditions, mental health issues, sleep disordered breathing, restless legs, and menopausal symptoms, and others as noted in Box 8.2. For example, snoring may be a clue to sleep apnea, and nocturia (urinary frequency overnight) may cause disrupted sleep or be a sign of sleep apnea (See also Chapter 11). A physical exam should focus on medical conditions that may cause difficulty sleeping, such as body mass index and enlarged tonsils for sleep apnea; changes in hair, nails, skin, eyes, or tremors for thyroid disorders; jugular venous pulsation, cardiac exam, lung exam, and evaluating extremities for swelling to evaluate for signs of congestive heart failure. If dementia or cognitive impairment is suspected, patients should be evaluated with an appropriate office screening tool such as the Mini-Cog.

Once conditions that may contribute to insomnia have been ruled out or mitigated, a sleep history will help to classify the sleep problems. The sleep history should include sleep quality, sleep latency and total time in bed (which allows

**Box 8.3 Common Terminology for Insomnia**

| | |
|---|---|
| Sleep quality | Overall satisfaction with the sleep experience |
| Sleep latency | Amount of time it takes to go from fully awake to asleep |
| Total sleep time (TST) | Time during a total sleep episode minus time awake, which includes tossing and turning |
| Time in bed (TIB) | The total time in bed, including time asleep and any time spent awake in bed (reading, texting, lying awake in bed) |
| Sleep efficiency (SE) | Percentage of time asleep while in bed (TST/TIB × 100). Please see section "Sleep Restriction (SR)" for an example |
| Wake after sleep onset (WASO) | A period of being awake after the initial sleep onset |
| Sleep window | Defined by TST and the patient's preference for going to bed and schedule demands |

calculation of sleep efficiency), wake after sleep onset (WASO), and the desired sleep window. It is also important to assess caffeine use, naps, and the bedroom environment (temperature, television use, etc.). You can find information about where to download sleep logs in Box 8.10.

> **Case (Continued)**
> **Martha's Sleep History**
> Martha gets up at 7 am for work. She usually goes to bed at 10 pm, but often has difficulty falling asleep and does not fall asleep until midnight. She wakes up twice per night and needs about 30 min to fall asleep again each time. She completed the sleep diary located here: http://sleepeducation.org/docs/default-document-library/sleep-diary.pdf
>
>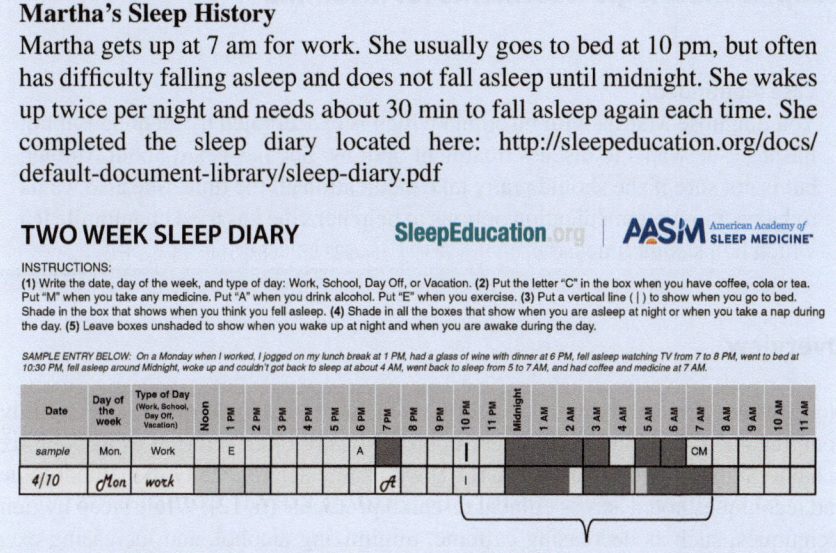
>
> Sleep diary from http://sleepeducation.org and used with permission from the American Academy of Sleep Medicine
>
> Time in bed (TIB): 9 h (10–7)
> Martha's total sleep time (TST) is only 6 h, since it takes her 2 h to fall asleep and she is awake for 1 h overnight. Her sleep efficiency (SE) is 6 h/9 h × 100 = 67%.

Normal sleep efficiency is 80% or greater. In Martha's case, her decreased sleep efficiency is caused both by an increased sleep latency and by her nighttime awakenings.

For evaluation of insomnia, the American Academy of Sleep Medicine (AASM) recommends the following [4]:

1. A general medical/psychiatric questionnaire to identify comorbid disorders
2. The Epworth Sleepiness Scale to identify issues with daytime sleepiness
3. A 2-week sleep log to identify general patterns of sleep–wake times and day-to-day variability

The AASM gives a conditional recommendation to the use of actigraphy, which is the use of a wrist or ankle monitor to measure movement during sleep. Actigraphy can be useful to evaluate sleep–wake and circadian rhythm disorders, especially when information from the sleep log is inconsistent or unclear. This is different from polysomnography (also known as a sleep study), which measures multiple parameters including brain waves, oxygenation, heart rate, respiratory rate, eye movements, and leg movements. Polysomnography and laboratory testing are not recommended for the routine evaluation of insomnia [4].

## Nonpharmacologic Treatments for Insomnia

> **Case (Continued)**
> You diagnose Martha with insomnia which is exacerbated by menopausal hot flashes. She wants to discuss treatment options. She has heard about Ambien but is not sure if she should really take medication all the time. She also wants to know about nonmedication options to help her. She has tried chamomile tea which helps sometimes.

## Overview

Nonpharmacological treatments incorporate educational, behavioral, and cognitive components. Combinations of these approaches are often referred to as cognitive behavioral therapy for insomnia (CBT-I) with some heterogeneity in methodologies and techniques noted across clinical research protocols [6, 12]. While sleep hygiene techniques, such as decreasing caffeine, minimizing alcohol, and increasing exercise, have minimal associated risk, they are less likely to be effective for patients with insomnia as opposed to occasional sleeplessness [31, 33–35].

Generally, CBT-I is a structured, time-bound approach that is recommended as the first-line treatment for insomnia [5, 7]. Common components of CBT-I include education, treatment rationale, symptom tracking, behavioral and cognitive components, and problem solving (Fig. 8.1) . Although initially developed for the treatment of *primary insomnia*, CBT-I has shown effectiveness for *secondary insomnia* with associated psychiatric and medical conditions such as alcohol use disorders, depression, PTSD, chronic pain, (breast) cancer, hearing impairment, chronic obstructive pulmonary disease (COPD), and osteoarthritis [8]. CBT-I is associated with significant improvements in sleep efficiency, quality, and sleep onset latency, while decreasing

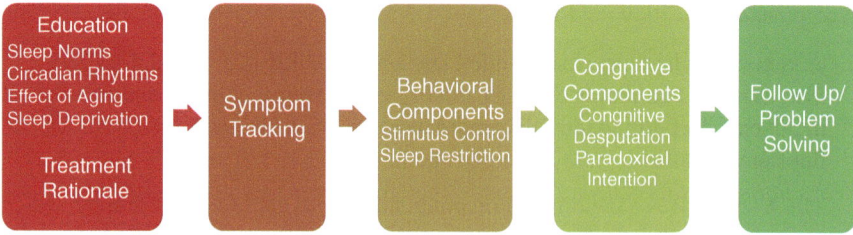

**Fig. 8.1** Common components of CBT-I

awakenings with smallest effect noted on the total sleep time [6]. Therapy can be delivered in various formats such as individual, group, phone, or online.

Evidence supporting digital delivery of CBT-I has been growing, with reported large short-term effects and ongoing (albeit smaller) effects for up to 18 months [26] and utility across diverse populations [27, 28]. However, further research is needed to better understand the mechanisms, dissemination, as well as limitations including higher dropout rates and limited tailoring to address patients' needs [28, 29].

Techniques of CBT-I aim to deepen and consolidate sleep, promote regular sleep patterns, elicit and support psychogenic relaxation response, and correct maladaptive sleeping thoughts and behaviors [9].

## Components of Cognitive Behavioral Therapy for Insomnia

### Education
Education links pretreatment evaluation to the intervention and provides education to develop realistic sleep expectations and to correct common misconceptions about sleep norms, circadian rhythms, aging, and sleep deprivation. Several age-related sleep changes have been outlined by the National Sleep Foundation (2003) including the following:

1. Changes in sleep architecture: decrease in rapid eye movement (REM) sleep, earlier bed and wake up times, decreased SE as the sleep becomes more fragmented.
2. Increased sensitivity to environmental disruptions (e.g., temperature), hormonal changes (e.g., menopause-related), and physical conditions (e.g., cancer)

For further information concerning sleep education as outlined in CBT-I, please refer to work of Hunter and colleagues [29] and *Overcoming Insomnia: A Cognitive Behavioral Therapy Approach* by Edinger and Carney [30]. It needs to be noted that CBT-I protocols do not specifically focus on the needs of either older or female patient populations.

### Symptom Tracking
Symptom tracking allows for the review of current sleep patterns and coping behaviors, as well as the assessment of patient's total sleep time (TST), wake after sleep onset (WASO), time in bed (TIB), sleep window, and sleep efficiency (SE) (please refer back to Box 8.3). Symptom tracking is used to guide interventions and make adjustments throughout treatment. The patient should complete at least a 2-week sleep log at baseline. Resources to access sleep logs are provided at the end of this chapter (see Box 8.10, Patient Handouts and Resources).

### Behavioral Components

### Stimulus Control (SC)
Developed by R. Bootzin, stimulus control is based on classical (Pavlovian) conditioning. SC aims to "strengthen the cues of bed and bedroom for sleep and

weakening the cues for activities that interfere with falling asleep" [10]. Activities and mental acts, such as reading, watching tv, worrying, which are done in bed, are viewed as "competing with sleep" as these weaken associations between bed and sleep. SC therapy has been effective as monotherapy or as a part of multicomponent CBT interventions. Box 8.4 lists behaviors that achieve SC.

Of note, to limit awake time in bed, the patient is specifically advised to leave the bed if she is unable to fall asleep in 10–20 min and/or becomes frustrated with her inability to fall asleep. She is advised to get up and go to another room until she begins to feel sleepy again. Generally, she is instructed to stay awake for at least 15 min before returning to the bedroom. During this time, she should not engage in any stimulating activities and should avoid screen time. This step is repeated as often as needed throughout the night.

### Sleep Restriction (SR)

Based on the work of A. Spielman, sleep restriction has been described as "systematic, controlled, partial form of sleep deprivation designed to consolidate sleep rapidly and then gradually increase the scheduled time allotted for sleep when adequate sleep efficiency has been achieved" [11]. Stand-alone SR is an effective treatment for improvement of core insomnia symptoms [12, 13] with improvements maintained at 3-month follow-up [12]. Literature reviews outline SR among other nonpharmacological treatments in older adults. Box 8.5 lists specific steps for SR. Important warnings and considerations that are outlined in Box 8.6 should be discussed in detail with the patient prior to recommending SR. Shared decision-making is very important for patient safety and success of the treatment.

---

**Box 8.4 Behaviors to Achieve Stimulus Control**
1. Limit bedroom activities to sleep and sex only.
2. Limit awake time in bed.
3. Only go to bed when already feeling sleepy.
4. Keep the same wake up time 7 days of the week.
5. Avoid daytime naps. However, for elderly patients, a brief (30 min) daytime nap can be scheduled. The specifics of the nap time and duration should be determined in collaboration with the patient.

---

**Case (Continued)**
Recall that Martha spends 9 h in bed every day and sleeps for only 6 h, for a sleep efficiency of 67%. She needs to get up at 7 am for work. She agrees to get up at the same time on the weekend. You ask Martha to go to bed at 1 am and get up at 7 am. This will ensure that she is only in bed as long as she currently sleeps. She should not nap during the day, but if she feels very sleepy during the day, she can go to bed at 12:45. Martha can go to bed 20 min earlier every week, as long as she maintains a sleep efficiency of at least 85%.

> **Box 8.5 Sleep Restriction Instructions**
> - Provide education, ensure patient is in agreement and understands the risks and benefits of SR.
> - Assess SE, TIB, sleep window.
> - Agree on a daily wake-up time.
> - Instruct patient to go to bed based on the current sleep window and get up at a set wake-up time.
> - Avoid daytime naps.
> - Continue tracking: once SE reaches 85%, increase time in bed by 15–20 min every week.

> **Box 8.6 Sleep Restriction (SR) Warnings and Considerations**
> - SR is *not appropriate* for patients suffering from: excessive daytime somnolence, neurologic conditions such as seizure disorders, non-REM parasomnias, and bipolar disorder. Sleep deprivation in these conditions may lead to increased distress, impairment, and/or decompensation.
> - Specifics of SR methodology *vary significantly across research trials* [13].
> - Before attempting SR, review the literature. Kyle and colleagues offer a good overview of the differences in SR therapy procedures [12].
> - Research indicates that patients undergoing SR have *significant impairments on the vigilance tasks throughout the treatment course of 4 weeks* [12].

## Cognitive Components

### Cognitive Disputation

Patient's thoughts and beliefs can act as antecedent and/or maintaining factors of sleep difficulties. Specific thinking patterns, although possibly rooted in facts, can lead to significant distress incompatible with state of relaxation required for sleep (Box 8.7). The goal of cognitive disputation is to help the patients interpret their own thoughts as hypotheses rather than facts and in doing so, reduce distress and promote coping.

> Patient's thoughts can be elicited using a question: "What is going through your mind when you cannot sleep?"

### Box 8.7 Common Thinking Patterns Associated with Distress

Common thinking patterns associated with distress

| Term | Description | Example |
|---|---|---|
| Jumping to conclusions | Making a negative interpretation despite of definite facts supporting it | My bad mood/work problems are all because I did not get enough sleep |
| All or nothing thinking | Seeing the situation in black-and/or-white terms. There are no compromises | If I cannot get 8 h of sleep, my whole day will be ruined |
| Self-fulfilling prophecy | Anticipate bad outcomes and treat predictions as facts | Because I was not able to fall asleep at night, I will not be able to get anything done today |
| Catastrophizing | Predicting the worst possible outcome | I am going to develop a serious health issue/die early because I cannot sleep |

Adapted from [29, 30]

Once patient's thoughts are identified, these are examined together with the patient. Remember, that the goal is *not* to argue the patient out of her current thinking but rather help her examine evidence for and against her beliefs, developing a thought or belief that is less distressing to the patient. Example of a cognitive disputation form is found in Box 8.8.

### Box 8.8 Sample Cognitive Disputation Form

| Situation | Mood | Thought | Evidence supporting my thought | Evidence not supporting my thought | New thought, including evidence supporting and not supporting first thought | Current mood |
|---|---|---|---|---|---|---|
| I'm at home, in bed, at 2 am, and I'm awake | Worried, frustrated, heart racing | If I don't get good sleep, my health will deteriorate and I will die. | My doctor told me sleep is important to my health. My mom also had insomnia and she died. | I am in good health even though I have insomnia. My mom didn't die from her insomnia. | Sleep is important for my health, and I want to work on getting better sleep, but insomnia will not kill me. | Less worried, less frustrated, heart rate back to normal. |

Adapted from [29, 30]

## Paradoxical Intention

Paradoxical intention is a prescriptive technique that instructs the patient to engage in feared or avoided behavior. For example, the patient who is afraid of not being able to fall asleep will be asked to go to bed and make an effort to stay awake. The paradoxical intention aims to decrease sleep-related performance anxiety leading to a fewer difficulties with sleep initiation. Paradoxical intention (as well as relaxation training for insomnia) was the common component in CBT-I research published in the 1970s; however, paradoxical intention is not frequently found in more recent CBT-I research protocols [6].

### Follow-Up

Within mental health settings, CBT-I is delivered within 4–10, weekly, hour-long sessions by a therapist (Substance Abuse and Mental Health Administration, 2018) [32]. Additionally, there is limited understanding of the CBT-I-related adherence and patient-specific factors. Specifically, we do not know the best patient profile for CBT-I and cannot be sure about dose–response relationship between symptom improvement and CBT-I techniques. With the emergence of online and app-based CBT-I, these questions are yet to be answered. CBT-I should be performed by providers who are familiar with the CBT techniques and principles or those who receive adequate supervision by a qualified professional.

## Other Nonpharmacologic Techniques

### Sleep Hygiene Education

Sleep hygiene instructions have limited utility for patients with chronic insomnia and may be better suited for patients with occasional sleep difficulties or those with poor sleep environments. Overall, while principles of good sleep hygiene should be followed by all, there is insufficient evidence to support sleep hygiene as an effective, stand-alone intervention for insomnia [5].

Sleep hygiene, also known as "good sleep habits," consists of behaviors, practices, and habits that may promote good sleep. The National Sleep Foundation outlines the following strategies for improvement of sleep hygiene: limiting daytime naps to 30 min; avoiding stimulants (caffeine, nicotine) close to bedtime; regularly exercising; avoiding foods that can be disruptive to sleep by producing indigestion; ensuring natural exposure to sunlight; establishing a relaxing nighttime routine; creating a pleasant sleep environment. Sleep hygiene instructions also frequently incorporate elements of sleep restriction or stimulus control strategies.

### Relaxation Training

Relaxation techniques such as progressive muscle relaxation and diaphragmatic breathing can create conditions of physical and cognitive relaxation which are necessary for sleep. Regular practice of relaxation training is needed to ensure success. Additionally, practitioners should be aware of the *paradoxical anxiety*—increase in cognitive, physiological, or behavioral anxiety components in response to systematic relaxation training [14]. It has been reported that progressive muscle relaxation may be associated with less paradoxical anxiety compared to other relaxation techniques [14].

| | |
|---|---|
| Relaxation apps | CBT-i Coach by US Department of Veterans Affairs (VA) |
| | Insomnia Coach by Palo Alto Veterans Institute for Research |
| | Sleep Cycle: smart alarm clock [26] |
| | Sleep as Android Unlock [26] |
| | Sleep Center Free [26] |
| | Good Morning Alarm Clock [26] |

## Biofeedback

Biofeedback is a group of therapeutic procedures whereby physiological functions such as heart rate, electrodermal activity, electroencephalogram (EEG), breathing, and others are measured, recorded, and transmitted to the patient via auditory or visual feedback. The patient is taught to develop awareness and voluntary control of these functions [15]. Utilization of biofeedback in insomnia treatment is controversial. Two recent review studies highlight methodological concerns in biofeedback research studies for insomnia calling for further randomized clinical trials (RCT) of higher methodological quality [16, 17].

## Additional Considerations

Heterogeneity of methods within CBT-I components and some overlaps between nonpharmacological techniques (e.g., use of SR in sleep hygiene) can be confusing for both physicians and patients. As with any lifestyle intervention, shared decision-making with the patient is critical to ensure safety and success.

# Pharmacotherapy Treatments for Insomnia

### Case (Continued)
You see Martha for a follow-up in 3 months and she has been working with a therapist using manualized CBT-I treatment. You note there is improvement in her symptoms but she continues to have delayed sleep onset two to three times per week. She is interested in discussing medication options.

There are several classes of medications commonly used to treat insomnia. Some of these medications are FDA-approved for insomnia, while many are used off label for their sedating properties. In older adults, benzodiazepines are potentially harmful and should generally be avoided if possible. These agents have decreased metabolism and increased sensitivity in older patients resulting in significant side effects such as cognitive dysfunction and falls which can result in fractures and motor vehicle accidents [23]. Box 8.9 lists classes of medications used in the treatment of insomnia and important points to keep in mind regarding each class of drugs.

**Box 8.9 Sedative-Hypnotics for Insomnia [24, 36]**

| | | |
|---|---|---|
| Benzodiazepine receptor agonists Nonbenzodiazepine drugs | Zaleplon Zolpidem Eszopiclone | *Side effects*: Morning sedation Anterograde amnesia Anxiety Impaired balance and falls Complex sleep-related behaviors (sleepwalking, sleep-related eating, driving, and sexual behavior) |
| Benzodiazepine receptor agonists Benzodiazepine drugs | Triazolam Temazepam Estazolam Flurazepam Alprazolam Lorazepam Clonazepam | *Generally avoid or use with extreme caution* in older patients due to increased risk of cognitive impairment and falls Risk for addiction and dependence Avoid with alcohol Avoid in patients with hepatic impairment Avoid in patients with untreated sleep apnea and respiratory failure |
| Melatonin agonists | Melatonin Ramelteon | Generally well tolerated with a few adverse effects |
| Sedating antidepressants | Doxepin Nortriptyline Trazodone Mirtazapine | *Side effects*: Orthostatic hypotension Anticholinergic side effects Cardiac conduction delay Mirtazapine: increased appetite and weight gain |
| Sedating antipsychotics | Olanzapine Quetiapine | *Side effects*: Weight gain and metabolic syndrome Dizziness Extrapyramidal symptoms Hypotension |
| Antihistamines | Diphenhydramine Doxylamine | *Side effects*: Anticholinergic Dystonia Urinary retention |
| Anticonvulsants | Gabapentin Pregabalin | *Side effects*: Ataxia Renally excreted: caution in patients with renal disease |
| Orexin receptor antagonists | Suvorexant Lemborexant | *Side effects*: Somnolence Headache Generally well tolerated with mild SEs in patients >65 years old; low risk of postural instability and falls |

For patients without contraindications, we recommend starting with Ramelteon, an FDA-approved melatonin agonist that is generally well tolerated with a few side effects.

When selecting medications for the treatment of insomnia, it is important to consider the side effect profile, cost, onset, and duration of action, and if there are any secondary effects of the medications that may be beneficial for the patient. It is important to employ shared decision-making and engage in a conversation that reviews the risks, benefits, and alternatives to pharmacotherapy.

It can be helpful to consider comorbidities when choosing medications for the treatment of insomnia. Patients suffering with coexisting depression may be offered a nighttime sedating antidepressant for the management of both insomnia and mood symptoms. Patients with chronic pain may benefit from amitriptyline, a sedating antidepressant that can also be used for treating pain syndromes. A patient suffering from peripheral neuropathy might find gabapentin or pregabalin relieves both their neuropathic pain and insomnia. An elderly patient with dementia and decreased appetite or weight loss may benefit from mirtazapine.

## Herbals and Supplements for Insomnia

The use of herbals and supplements is very common among patients over the age of 50. Based on 2007 survey statistics from the National Center for Complementary and Integrative Health, approximately 40% of US adults over the age of 50 use complementary and alternative medicines (CAM) [17]. Another national survey done in 2010 demonstrated that a striking 67% of those using CAM did not discuss their use with their health care providers [18]. Patients often combine prescription medications with herbals and supplements without fully understanding risks of drug–herb/supplement interactions. In fact, 26% of patients over the age of 50 who used CAM were taking two to three prescription medications [18]. It is important to ask patients about CAM use before prescribing any medications for insomnia to ensure safety and avoid harmful interactions.

> *A Word of Caution!*
> Over-the-counter supplements are not regulated by the Food and Drug Administration (FDA). Patients should be cautioned that some supplement products contain possibly harmful impurities or additives. Patients should be advised to check with a pharmacist for more details regarding the particular brand they choose to use. Brands that have been vetted by third party organizations, confirming that the company practices good manufacturing practices, are safest if patients opt to try over-the-counter supplements.

Commonly used herbals and supplements for insomnia include valerian root, chamomile, melatonin, hops, passionflower, and lemon balm. It is important to note that herbals and supplements are not FDA approved, and generally the evidence for effectiveness, quality, and safety is inconsistent. Further studies are needed to make strong recommendations regarding the use of herbals and supplements for insomnia. For patients who are interested in herbals/supplements for insomnia and sleep quality, the following can be recommended given their favorable safety profiles. It is important to keep in mind that any herbal/supplement that has sedative effects should be used with extreme caution with medications that are used for insomnia (particularly benzodiazepines) as the combination can exacerbate adverse effects. They should also be avoided with concomitant alcohol use.

## Chamomile

A recent systematic review and meta-analysis of RCTs evaluated the therapeutic efficacy and safety of chamomile for insomnia and sleep quality and concluded that chamomile appears to be safe and effective for improving sleep quality. However, larger RCTs are needed to support these findings [19]. Patients can choose to try either one cup of chamomile tea or capsule with 220 mg flower standardized to contain 1.2% apigenin before bed.

## Melatonin

Aging is associated with both dysfunction in circadian rhythms and a reduction in melatonin levels, especially as women approach menopause. These factors play an important role in the commonly experienced peri- and postmenopausal sleep problems. Studies have shown that exogenous melatonin supplementation may improve sleep latency and quality at low doses with a few adverse effects and drug–supplement interactions, although further studies are required to make strong recommendations [20]. Patients can try 2–3 mg of sublingual or oral immediate-release (for sleep onset) or sustained-release (for sleep maintenance) melatonin supplements as needed at bedtime.

## Valerian Root

A randomized placebo-controlled trial studied the effect of valerian root extract on sleep quality in postmenopausal women aged 50–60 years old. Valerian root improved sleep quality in women with menopause and the study supported its use in the clinical management of insomnia [21]. Other studies have shown that valerian modestly reduces sleep latency by approximately 15 min and improves subjective sleep quality. Continuous nightly dosing of 400–900 mg of valerian root for several days up to 4 weeks may be necessary for therapeutic benefits [22].

> **Case (Continued)**
>
> After discussing the medication options and their side effects with Martha, she chooses to try over the counter melatonin supplements because her insurance does not cover ramelteon. Because of her relatively young age and low risk of falls, you also prescribe zolpidem to use as needed if the melatonin does not work. You use the teach-back technique to confirm you adequately explained that she does not combine melatonin and zolpidem together and she has to avoid alcohol when using these treatments. You obtain Martha's written permission to speak with her CBT-I therapist to help you with care coordination.
>
> You also discuss with Martha that treatment of her hot flashes may also help in the management of her insomnia. You explain that some women find using fans or keeping their room temperature low can be helpful though there is little scientific evidence that these interventions work. The most effective treatment is hormone replacement therapy with estrogen, followed by nonestrogen medications such as antidepressants, gabapentin, pregabalin, and clonidine. Paced respirations which are slow, deep, diaphragmatic breathing exercises can also be an effective nonpharmacotherapy option for managing hot flashes.
>
> Martha has heard that hormones can cause blood clots and cancer. You assure her that hormone therapy is safe in appropriately selected patients (See also Chapter 11). She expresses she would rather try the nonmedication options you taught her first and will cut out the wine in the evenings to see if that helps. You offer her some helpful handouts and web-based resources while also setting up a follow up visit in 1 month.

**Box 8.10 Resources for Patients**

| | |
|---|---|
| Apps | CBT-i Coach by US Department of Veterans Affairs (VA) |
| | Insomnia Coach by Palo Alto Veterans Institute for Research |
| | Sleep Cycle: smart alarm clock [25] |
| | Sleep as Android Unlock [25] |
| | Sleep Center Free [25] |
| | Good Morning Alarm Clock [25] |

| | |
|---|---|
| Patient Handouts and Resources | Sleep Changes in Older Adults from Family Doctor: https://familydoctor.org/sleep-changes-in-older-adults/<br>Healthy Sleep Tips for Women from National Sleep Foundation: https://www.sleepfoundation.org/articles/healthy-sleep-tips-women<br>Patient Facts: Insomnia from American College of Physicians https://www.acponline.org/system/files/documents/practice-resources/patient-resources/insomnia-facts.pdf<br>Sleep Self Care from University of California, Berkley: https://uhs.berkeley.edu/sites/default/files/insomnia.pdf<br>Sleep Diary from National Sleep Foundation: https://www.sleepfoundation.org/sites/default/files/inline-files/sample_sleep_log-by_national_sleep_foundation.pdf<br>Sleep Diary from AASM: http://sleepeducation.org/docs/default-document-library/sleep-diary.pdf |
| Websites | National Sleep Foundation https://www.sleepfoundation.org/<br>Relaxation Exercise from National Sleep Foundation: https://www.sleepfoundation.org/insomnia/treatment/relaxation-exercise<br>Drweil.com: Natural Insomnia Treatment https://www.drweil.com/health-wellness/body-mind-spirit/sleep-issues/natural-insomnia-treatment/<br>Free Cognitive Behavioral Therapy for Insomnia http://freecbti.com/ |
| Books | Hunter et al. [29]<br>Edinger and Carney [30] |

# References

1. Maness DL, Khan M. Nonpharmacologic management of chronic insomnia. Am Fam Physician. 2015;92(12):1058–64.
2. American Psychiatric Association. Diagnostic and statistical manual of mental disorders. 5th ed. Washington, DC: American Psychiatric Association; 2013.
3. Satela MJ. International classification of sleep disorders. Third edition. Chest. 2014;146(5):1387–94.
4. Winkelman JW. Insomnia disorder. N Engl J Med. 2015;373:1437–44.
5. Schutte-Rodin S, Broch L, Buysse D, Dorsey C, Sateia M. Clinical guideline for the evaluation and management of chronic insomnia in adults. J Clin Sleep Med. 2008;4(5):487–504.
6. van Straten A, van der Zweerde T, Kleiboer A, Cuijpers P, Morin CM, Lancee J. Cognitive and behavioral therapies in the treatment of insomnia: a meta-analysis. Sleep Med Rev. 2018;38:3–16. https://doi.org/10.1016/j.smrv.2017.02.001.
7. Qaseem A, Kansagara D, Forciea MA, Cooke M, Denberg TD. Clinical Guidelines Committee of the American College of Physicians. Management of chronic insomnia disorder in adults:

8. Wu JQ, Appleman ER, Salazar RD, Ong JC. Cognitive behavioral therapy for insomnia comorbid with psychiatric and medical conditions: a meta-analysis. JAMA Intern Med. 2015;175(9):1461–72.
9. Buenaver LF, Townsend D, Ong JC. Delivering cognitive behavioral therapy for insomnia in the real world: considerations and controversies. Sleep Med. 2019;14(2):275–81.
10. Bootzin RR, Perlis ML. Stimulus control therapy. In: Behavioral treatments for sleep disorders. 2011. p. 21–30. Available from: https://www.med.upenn.edu/cbti/assets/user-content/documents/btsd%2D%2Dstimuluscontrol-bsmtxprotocols.pdf
11. Sharma MP, Andrade C. Behavioral interventions for insomnia: theory and practice. Indian J Psychiatry. 2012;54(4):359–66. https://doi.org/10.4103/0019-5545.104825.
12. Kyle SD, Aquino MR, Miller CB, Henry AL, Crawford MR, Espie CA, Spielman AJ. Towards standardisation and improved understanding of sleep restriction therapy for insomnia disorder: a systematic examination of CBT-I trial content. Sleep Med Rev. 2015;23:83–8. https://doi.org/10.1016/j.smrv.2015.02.003.
13. Miller CB, Espie CA, Epstein DR, Friedman L, Morin CM, Pigeon WR, Spielman AJ, Kyle SD. The evidence base of sleep restriction therapy for treating insomnia disorder. Sleep Med Rev. 2014;18(5):415–24. https://doi.org/10.1016/j.smrv.2014.01.006.
14. Heide FJ, Borkovec TD. Relaxation-induced anxiety: paradoxical anxiety enhancement due to relaxation training. J Consult Clin Psychol. 1983;51(2):171–82.
15. Melo DLM, Carvalho LBC, Prado LBF, Prado GF. Biofeedback therapies for chronic insomnia: a systematic review. Appl Psychophysiol Biofeedback. 2019;44(4):259–69. https://doi.org/10.1007/s10484-019-09442-2.
16. Lovato N, Miller CB, Gordon CJ, Grunstein RR, Lack L. The efficacy of biofeedback for the treatment of insomnia: a critical review. Sleep Med. 2019;56:192–200. https://doi.org/10.1016/j.sleep.2018.12.011.
17. Barnes PM, Bloom B, Nahin R. Complementary and alternative medicine use among adults and children: United States, 2007. CDC National Health Statistics Reports #12.
18. AARP, NCCAM. Complementary and alternative medicine: what people aged 50 and older discuss with their health care providers. Consumer Survey Report; April 13, 2010.
19. Hieu TH, Dibas M, Surya Dila KA, Sherif NA, Hashmi MU, Mahmoud M, Trang NTT, Abdullah L, Nghia TLB, Hirayama K, Huy NT. Therapeutic efficacy and safety of chamomile for state anxiety, generalized anxiety disorder, insomnia, and sleep quality: a systematic review and meta-analysis of randomized trials and quasi-randomized trials. Phytother Res. 2019;33(6):1604–15.
20. Jehan S, Jean-Louis G, Zizi F, Auguste E, Pandi-Perumal SR, Gupta R, Attarian H, McFarlane SI, Hardeland R, Brzezinski A. Sleep, melatonin, and the menopausal transition: what are the links? Sleep Sci. 2017;10(1):11–8.
21. Taavoni S, Ekbatani N, Kashaniyan M, Haghani H. Effect of valerian on sleep quality in postmenopausal women: a randomized placebo-controlled clinical trial. Menopause. 2011;18(9):951–5.
22. Natural Medicines. Valerian Root [Monograph]. Natural Standard Professional Monograph; 2019, February 12. Retrieved from https://naturalmedicines.therapeuticresearch.com/databases/food,-herbs-supplements/professional.aspx?productid=870#scientificName
23. 2019 American Geriatrics Society Beers Criteria® Update Expert Panel. American Geriatrics Society 2019 updated AGS beers criteria® for potentially inappropriate medication use in older adults. J Am Geriatr Soc. 2019;67(4):674–94.
24. Buysse DJ. Insomnia. JAMA. 2013;309(7):706–16. https://doi.org/10.1001/jama.2013.193.
25. Choi YK, Demiris G, Lin SY, et al. Smartphone applications to support sleep self-management: review and evaluation. J Clin Sleep Med. 2018;14(10):1783–90. Published 2018 Oct 15.

26. Luik AI, van der Zweerde T, van Straten A, Lancee J. Digital delivery of cognitive behavioral therapy for insomnia. Curr Psychiatry Rep. 2019;21(7):50. https://doi.org/10.1007/s11920-019-1041-0.
27. van der Zweerde T, Lancee J, Ida Luik A, van Straten A. Internet-delivered cognitive behavioral therapy for insomnia: tailoring cognitive behavioral therapy for insomnia for patients with chronic insomnia. Sleep Med Clin. 2019;14(3):301–15. https://doi.org/10.1016/j.jsmc.2019.04.002.
28. Drerup ML, Ahmed-Jauregui S. Online delivery of cognitive behavioral therapy-insomnia: considerations and controversies. Sleep Med Clin. 2019;14(2):283–90. https://doi.org/10.1016/j.jsmc.2019.02.001.
29. Hunter CL, Goodie JL, Oordt MS, Dobmeyer A. Integrated behavioral health in primary care: step-by-step guidance for assessment and intervention. Washington, DC: American Psychological Association; 2014.
30. Edinger JD, Carney CE. Overcoming insomnia: a cognitive-behavioral therapy approach, workbook. 2nd ed. Oxford: Oxford University Press; 2014.
31. National Sleep Foundation. Sleep and aging well; 2003. Retrieved from: http://www.sleepcenterofgreaterpittsburgh.com/downloads/sleep_aging_well.pdf
32. Substance Abuse and Mental Health Administration. Sleep and the eight dimensions. Cognitive behavioral therapy for insomnia (CBT-I); 2019. Retrieved from https://www.samhsa.gov/sites/default/files/programs_campaigns/wellness_initiative/cognitive-behavioral-therapy-for-insomnia-fact-sheet.pdf
33. Patel D, Steinberg J, Patel P. Insomnia in the elderly: a review. J Clin Sleep Med. 2018;14(6):1017–24.
34. Wennberg AM, Canham SL, Smith MT, Spira AP. Optimizing sleep in older adults: treating insomnia. Maturitas. 2013;76(3):247–52. https://doi.org/10.1016/j.maturitas.2013.05.007.
35. Brewster GS, Riegel B, Gehrman PR. Insomnia in the older adult. Sleep Med Clin. 2018;13(1):13–9. https://doi.org/10.1016/j.jsmc.2017.09.002.
36. Rosenberg R, Murphy P, Zammit G, et al. Comparison of Lemborexant with placebo and zolpidem tartrate extended release for the treatment of older adults with insomnia disorder: a phase 3 randomized clinical trial. JAMA Netw Open. 2019;2(12):e1918254. https://doi.org/10.1001/jamanetworkopen.2019.18254.

# Pelvic Organ Prolapse

## Christina Escobar and Dominique Malacarne Pape

**Key Points**
- Pelvic organ prolapse (POP) is relaxation of the vaginal walls that support the uterus, bladder, and rectum.
- POP is common and its prevalence increases with age, vaginal delivery, parity, and body mass index (BMI).
- POP symptoms may include a sensation of vaginal pressure or bulge and difficulty evacuating the bladder or rectum. Many women with POP are asymptomatic.
- Asymptomatic POP does not require treatment if a patient does not have urinary retention or hydronephrosis.
- Patients should be reassured that prolapse is not dangerous and it is safe to have sex with a prolapse; having sex will not make the prolapse worse.
- If bothered, patients with prolapse should be offered treatment: pelvic floor muscle exercises, a silicone support device (pessary), and surgery.
- For additional treatment, consider referral to a physical therapist for supervised pelvic floor muscle exercise training and to a urogynecologist (or gynecologist) for discussion of pessary and surgery options.

C. Escobar · D. Malacarne Pape (✉)
Department of Obstetrics and Gynecology,
New York University Medical Center, New York, NY, USA
e-mail: Christina.Escobar@nyulangone.org

**Case**

Sandy is a 63-year-old G3P3 who presents for an annual exam. She takes HCTZ 12.5 for hypertension and has never had surgery. She wants to talk about her weight, which has gradually crept up since menopause. She is having some right hip pain and thinks her weight is contributing. She is sexually active with her husband and does not report any issues. Her BMI is 32 and her physical exam is unremarkable. When you perform her pelvic exam to obtain a Pap smear, you note that her cervix is at the vaginal opening (Fig. 9.1). You tell Sandy that you see some relaxation of her vaginal walls, also called "prolapse," and ask whether she experiences any symptoms, such as feeling a bulge or sense of pressure, or difficulty starting or completing urination or bowel movements. You also ask about postmenopausal bleeding. She denies these symptoms but wants to know more about prolapse. Why does she have it?

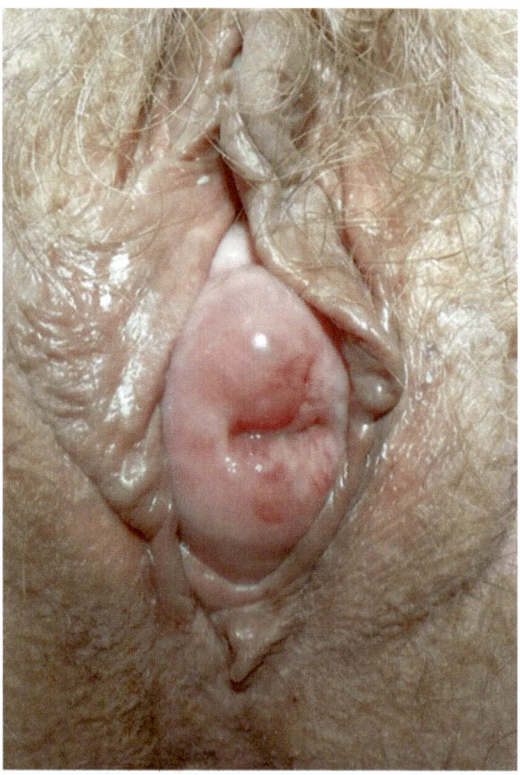

**Fig. 9.1** Pelvic organ prolapse on exam. (Info: By Mikael Häggström—Own work, CC0. https://commons.wikimedia.org/w/index.php?curid=36698443)

## Epidemiology

Pelvic organ prolapse is defined as the descent of anterior vaginal wall, posterior vaginal wall, apex of the vagina (cervix/uterus), or vaginal vault (cuff, after hysterectomy) [1]. Prolapse is commonly present in postmenopausal women, even in absence of symptoms. In a sub-analysis of the Women's Health Initiative (WHI) Hormone Replacement Therapy Clinical Trial, 41% of women had some degree of POP on physical exam [2]. However, the lifetime risk of symptomatic POP is lower. A cross-sectional national survey showed 2.9% (95% CI 2.5–3.4) of women reported symptomatic POP [3]. An analysis of US insurance claims and encounters database illustrated the lifetime risk for surgery for POP was 12.6% (95% CI 12.4, 12.7) [4]. As our population ages the total number of women who undergo surgery for POP is predicted to increase by 46% by 2050 [5]. The average annual cost of ambulatory care visits in the United States from 2005 to 2006 for the diagnosis of POP was 96.9 million dollars [6].

## Risk Factors

The etiology of POP is multifactorial [7–9]. Those risk factors most consistently citied in the literature are vaginal delivery, parity, age, and body mass index (BMI). Vaginal delivery, and in particular, operative delivery with forceps, is the most commonly identified risk factor for POP [10, 11]. Parity is also a clear risk factor for POP [2, 7, 12], with the risk of POP increasing with each child; however, the rate of increase declines after two children [12]. Another consistent factor associated with POP is age [2, 7]. The prevalence of POP increases by 40% with each decade [13]. In one study, in a managed care population, the largest number of consults for POP were for women in their 60s to 70s [14]. Finally, increased BMI is widely recognized to be a risk factor for POP. Several studies have shown that those who are overweight and obese are at higher risk of POP [2, 15]. In one meta-analysis, women who were overweight had a 40% increased risk of POP and women who were obese had a 50% increased risk of POP compared with normal weight peers [16]. BMI is also linked to an increased risk of having surgery for POP. One case-control study looking at risk factors for POP surgery showed that women with a BMI greater than 26 were more likely to have surgery for POP [10]. Of the risk factors with the strongest associations with POP in the literature, BMI is the only modifiable risk factor. Patients can be counseled on various options for weight reduction, as a way to prevent or improve POP symptoms, while also improving overall health and wellness. In a meta-analysis of the effects of bariatric surgery on pelvic floor disorders, weight loss via bariatric surgery resulted in an improvement in POP [17].

The epidemiologic associations with other potential POP risk factors are less clear. While patients and providers may commonly associate hysterectomy with a higher risk of POP, this association is controversial. The association between race and ethnicity and pelvic organ prolapse has been shown in some studies; however, the etiology for these differences is unclear [2]. In a cross-sectional study of women enrolled in the WHI, Hispanic women had a higher risk of POP compared to white women. A second study showed that compared with African-American women,

Hispanic and white women had four to five times higher risk of symptomatic prolapse, but other studies failed to detect this difference [19, 20].

The consensus in the literature regarding chronic strain on the pelvic floor and the risk of prolapse is even less clear. There are specific comorbidities that a patient might have which put strain on the pelvic floor, such as chronic cough, chronic obstructive pulmonary disease (COPD), and constipation. In one small observational study, constipation was more common in women with POP [18]. Several larger studies have refuted this [19–21]. It is also often thought that jobs with heavy lifting can strain the pelvic floor. In a case-control study of assistant nurses in Denmark, the risk of needing surgery for POP was higher among assistant nurses when compared to controls (OR = 1.6 (1.3–1.9), $P < 0.0001$). This led the authors to hypothesize that heavy lifting/activity at work led to the increased risk of POP [22]. Other studies have not found heavy physical activity to be a risk factor for POP [7].

## Pathophysiology

The pelvic organs are supported by both the levator ani muscles and connective tissue attachments (Fig. 9.2). These muscles and connective tissues support the openings of the vagina, urethra, and anus.

These muscles are contracted at rest and provide a floor for the pelvic organs to rest on. Muscle trauma can affect the tone of the pelvic floor and lead to a weakening of the levator ani and therefore POP can ensue. In patients with a history of vaginal deliveries, there can be visible defects in levator ani seen on MRI [23]. Furthermore, modeling has shown the levator ani to be stretched more than 200 times the threshold for stretch injuries during the second stage of labor [24].

The connective tissue attachments of the pelvic organs, also known as endopelvic fascia, are also essential for support. The condensation of the endopelvic fascia attaches the pelvic organs to the bones and muscles of the pelvis. These connective tissue attachments can be affected during child birth, hysterectomy, straining, or as a part of normal aging [25]. Additionally, those with connective tissue disorders may have a less robust support structure, which can lead to POP [26].

## Clinical Findings

### History

Taking a thorough history to screen for symptoms of POP and identify their associated bother is important, because POP can have a significant negative impact on quality of life [27–29]. Lack of knowledge of changes in pelvic floor function in the reproductive years can lead to lack of appropriate therapies as women age, causing unnecessary progression of disease.

The most common symptom of POP is vaginal pressure or a feeling of a bulge through the vaginal opening. A single simple screening question, "Do you have a bulge or something falling out that you can see or feel in your vaginal area?" has a sensitivity of 96% (95% CI 92–100) and specificity of 79% (95% CI 77–92) for

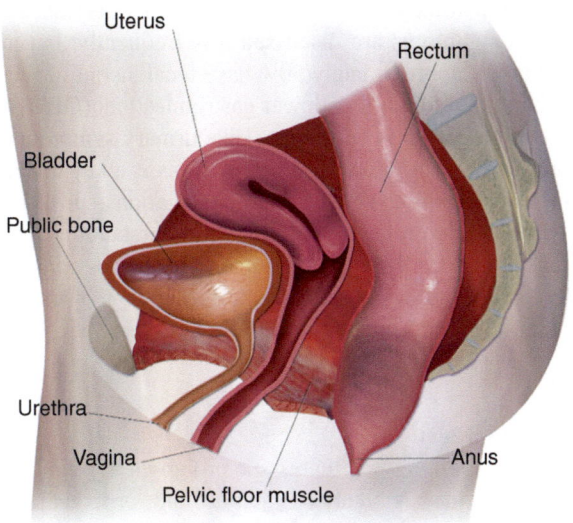

**Fig. 9.2** Female pelvic floor. (Info: Bruce Blaus/ CC-BY-SA-4.0. https:// commons.wikimedia.org/ wiki/File:Pelvic_Muscles_ (Female_Side).png)

Female Pelvic Muscles

prolapse at or beyond the hymen [30]. This question should be followed by further questioning and a physical exam to confirm the diagnosis.

> **Clinical Pearl**
> If a patient reports that her prolapse is interfering with penile penetration, it is important to ask about her partner's erections. While advanced prolapse can interfere with vaginal penetration, this symptom is more commonly a sign of erectile dysfunction and referral to urology may be helpful.

Bladder and bowel symptoms are very common in women with POP. While the symptoms of vaginal pressure, bulge, and even sexual dysfunction can be caused by prolapse itself, other symptoms can be caused by effect of prolapse on the bladder (urinary incontinence, voiding dysfunction) or the lower gastrointestinal (GI) tract (fecal incontinence or incomplete defecation). Of note, while bladder and/or bowel symptoms may be exacerbated by POP, they may be unrelated and co-occur with POP, so they should not be automatically attributed to POP.

In women with POP, 43% have stress urinary incontinence (SUI), 37% have overactive bladder and 29% have mixed incontinence [31]. It is thought that cystocele formation can damage the support system of the urethra and influence SUI [32, 33]. Conversely, urinary retention can occur in advanced prolapse due to urethral kinking. In one study, 30% of patients with stage III or greater prolapse had a post-void residual (PVR) of greater than 100 mL [34]. While it is easy to see how prolapse can affect urinary symptoms, it is important to remember that these symptoms can also be present regardless of POP status, as women without prolapse also develop urinary symptoms.

While urinary symptoms are commonly discussed in conjunction with prolapse, bowel symptoms are discussed less frequently, but are also prevalent. In women with POP, approximately 50% have fecal incontinence [31]. In patients with POP, it is important to work up lower gastrointestinal (GI) symptoms and ensure screening for colon cancer is up to date. Like urinary symptoms, defecatory disorders can be present in the absence of prolapse. This is a key concept for patients to understand in terms of prolapse treatment expectations. In trying to understand if lower GI symptoms are related to prolapse, understanding the chronology of symptoms is paramount. If GI symptoms came first it is possible that constipation or diarrhea (± hyperdefecation) can exacerbate prolapse. However, if prolapse symptoms came first, the altered anatomy in POP can, in turn, be the driving factor.

> **Clinical Pearl**
> If a patient reports that tissue prolapses through her anus rather than through her vagina, she likely has hemorrhoids or rectal prolapse, and the most appropriate referral is colorectal surgery, not urogynecology.

> **Case (Continued)**
> You explain to Sandy that her three vaginal deliveries, age, and BMI are likely reasons she has developed pelvic organ prolapse. She asks what additional tests she will need and how the prolapse can be treated. She is terrified of surgery.

## Physical

A comprehensive physical exam is essential in the care of patients with pelvic organ prolapse. Pulmonary and cardiac exams may identify risk factors important in the consideration of surgical management. An abdominal exam can screen for scars from previous surgeries not mentioned in the history and find masses that might alter the treatment plan.

Measurement of prolapse occurs during the vaginal exam, which should occur supine and with standing if the patient reports symptoms that do not correlate with supine exam findings. Measurement of prolapse should occur both at rest and with straining. The vaginal exam should begin with an inspection of the external genitalia as well as the vaginal mucosa. When defining prolapse, the vagina should be divided into three compartments: anterior compartment, posterior compartment, and apex (Fig. 9.3). Using anterior compartment, posterior compartment, and apex is preferred as opposed to cystocele, rectocele, and enterocele. This is because the location of the prolapse of the vaginal wall does not reliably predict the association of prolapse of the organ [35, 36].

Each compartment is distinct, and a patient can have prolapse in a single compartment or a combination of compartments. Apical prolapse refers to descent of the cervix or vaginal cuff (post-hysterectomy) to within 4 cm of the hymen. Anterior compartment prolapse is descent of the anterior vaginal wall proximal to the urethrovesical junction (about 3 cm from the urethral meatus). If the anterior vaginal wall descends toward or beyond the hymen with Valsalva, the patient has anterior vaginal wall prolapse. The anterior compartment is most common compartment to prolapse [2]. Similarly, prolapse of the posterior compartment is seen when the posterior vaginal wall descends toward or beyond the hymen with Valsalva. A bi-valved speculum (Fig. 9.4) can be separated and the bottom half can be used to aid in assessment of mobility and descent of the anterior and posterior vaginal walls in isolation.

There are various prolapse measurement systems; however, the POP-Q is the most common, and is the preferred measurement system to record the stage of prolapse [36–38]. The POP-Q is a 9 item assessment system of vaginal support that measures points on the surface of the vagina in relation to the hymen on maximal strain. The only value not measured on maximal strain is total vaginal length (Fig. 9.5). Patients should be asked to bear down or perform a Valsalva maneuver during these measurements. This is a useful tool for measuring prolapse in a universal language and is widely used by specialist providers.

After prolapse assessment, a specialist might then perform several additional exams to complete the work up. A bimanual exam could be done to look for pelvic masses or uterine tenderness. A focused neurologic exam can help rule out undiagnosed neurologic issues [39]. A rectal exam would also be useful in determining the extent of posterior wall prolapse as well as to assess for anal sphincter tone. In a patient with any symptoms concerning for urinary tract infection (UTI), a complete urinalysis and urine culture would be performed, as UTI can potentiate voiding dysfunction. Finally, in patients with symptoms of difficulty emptying their bladder or with prolapse beyond the hymen measuring a post-void residual (PVR) can help evaluate for incomplete bladder emptying.

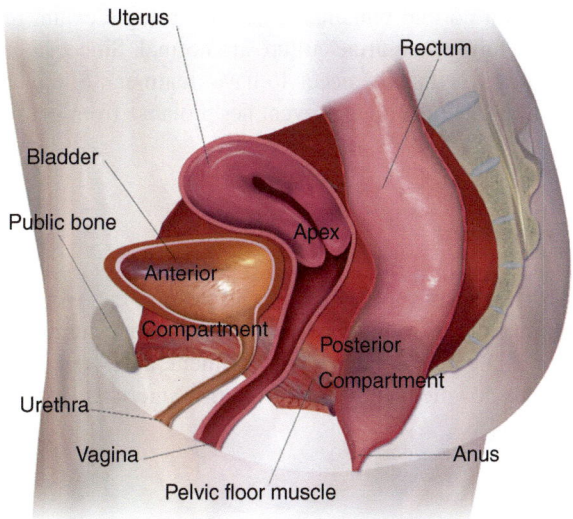

**Fig. 9.3** Compartments of the vagina. (Info: Bruce Blaus/CC-BY-SA-4.0. https://commons.wikimedia.org/wiki/File:Pelvic_Muscles_(Female_Side).png)

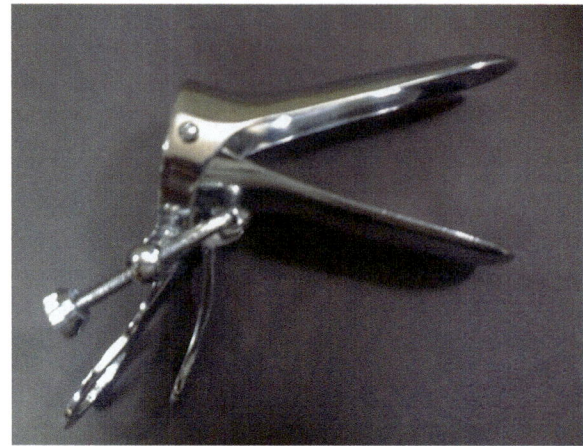

**Fig. 9.4** Bi-valved speculum. (Info: By Sarindam7—Own work, CC-BY-SA-4.0,3.0,2.5,2.0,1.0. https://commons.wikimedia.org/wiki/File:Cusco%27s_selfretaining_bivalve_vaginal_speculum_open.jpg)

## Additional Testing

There are various additional tests that can be performed in special cases. Urodynamic testing is typically reserved for uncovering other potential etiologies for elevated PVR or bothersome voiding symptoms [37]. Additionally, MRI defecography can be employed for cases of unusual prolapse anatomy, when symptoms do not correlate with exam or in women with incomplete bowel evacuation. These tests should be used judiciously and are commonly ordered by a female pelvic medicine and reconstructive surgery (FPMRS) or female urology specialist.

> **Case (Continued)**
> Sandy has both anterior and apical uterine prolapse based on your exam. She has a normal bimanual exam, neurologic exam, rectal exam and PVR. Her urinalysis and urine culture are normal. Since she has not had symptoms, she asks whether she needs to have treatment. She is also asking if there is anything she can do to prevent her prolapse from getting worse.

## Treatment

The treatment for POP varies and patients can work with providers to choose from a range of interventions, from conservative to surgical in nature. Providing information is a cornerstone of POP treatment, and we recommend these handouts, which can be downloaded for free from the American Urogynecologic Society.

1. Pelvic Organ Prolapse (https://www.voicesforpfd.org/assets/2/6/POP_Large_Print.pdf)
2. Pelvic Floor Muscle Exercises (https://www.voicesforpfd.org/assets/2/6/Bladder_Training_Large_Print.pdf)
3. Vaginal Pessaries (https://www.voicesforpfd.org/assets/2/6/Vaginal_Pessaries_Large_Print.pdf)
4. What is a Urogynecologist? (https://www.voicesforpfd.org/assets/2/6/What_is_a_Urogynecologist.pdf)

## Conservative Management

It is important to recognize that not all patients with pelvic organ prolapse require treatment. Asymptomatic patients usually do not require intervention. If the patient chooses to observe the potential progression of her prolapse, there are some important areas of consideration. First, the patient should present for periodic examination. These patients should be monitored closely for issues with urinary retention. Patients should be screened for symptoms of incomplete emptying and a post-void residual should be obtained. In patients who have an elevated PVR, imaging of the upper urinary tract with a renal ultrasound can help to diagnose the presence of hydronephrosis. Recurrent UTIs can be one sign of incomplete emptying, as urinary stasis leads to the overgrowth of bacteria. In order to monitor for recurrent UTIs, the provider should discuss any urinary tract infections that have happened since the last visit, as patients may present to an urgent care or may see other physicians for help with these symptoms. Additionally, patients should be monitored for severe

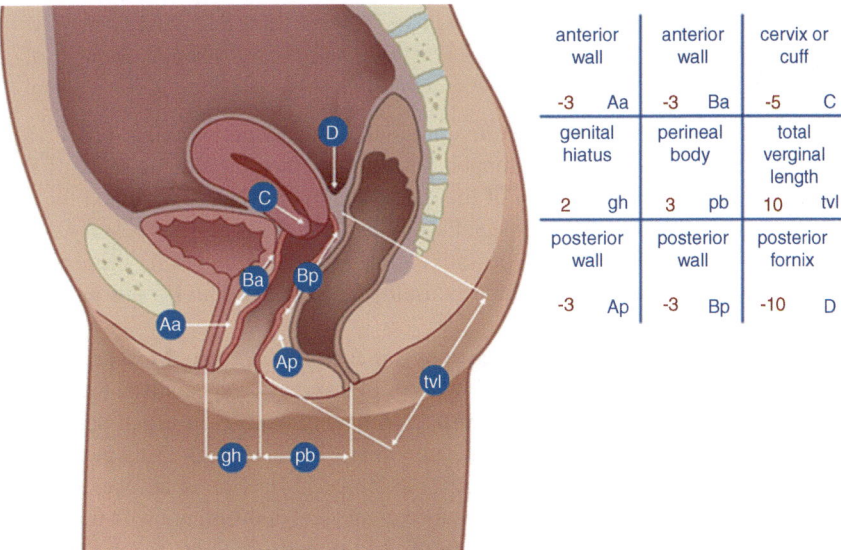

**Fig. 9.5** The POP-Q System: (Info by: https://www.augs.org/patient-services/pop-q-tool/)

vaginal or cervical erosions and obstructed defecation. All of the above conditions are considered contraindications to expectant management.

For the otherwise healthy asymptomatic patient with mild to moderate prolapse, these periodic assessments can occur in conjunction with the patient's yearly gynecological exam. The patient should be instructed to call and present sooner for evaluation if she becomes symptomatic. Occasionally patients with very advanced prolapse will present with no symptoms and desire observation. In these patients, evaluating bladder emptying is extremely important, and follow up every 3–6 months is recommended [40].

## Pelvic Floor Physical Therapy

A second conservative option that can be offered to women with POP is pelvic floor physical therapy (PFPT). This usually consists of at home exercises (Kegels) performed by the patient as guided by a formal physical therapy program with a physical therapist. It is paramount, if employing this modality, that patients understand expectations for time commitment and treatment duration. PFPT is more effective in improving symptoms of urinary incontinence than pelvic organ prolapse, but may provide some symptomatic improvement for prolapse [41]. While PFPT may slow progression of disease in those with severe prolapse, it is unlikely to result in improvement in POP-Q stage [41–43].

You can contact your hospital system's physical therapy department to learn whether there are physical therapists with pelvic floor training in your system. You can also visit www.apta.org and use the "Find a Provider" link to search for other physical therapists in your area.

## Pessary

The pessary is another conservative option for patients seeking relief from POP. There is good evidence to support pessary use for symptomatic relief of POP bother and health-related quality of life due to POP [44–51]. As an option for conservative management, 75% of specialists in the United States offer pessary as first line management of POP [52]. A pessary can also be placed by primary care providers or general gynecologists, which is useful for patients who do not have local access to specialists [53].

There are many available varieties of pessaries to choose from. Most are made of silicone and come in various sizes (Fig. 9.6). In a survey of specialists, there was a lack of defined practice patterns in respect to how to choose an initial pessary for each patient [52]. However in general, support pessaries, such as a ring pessary, are most commonly used in practice as a first choice [54]. This is an excellent first choice because of its simple design. Many patients feel comfortable with this design because it appears similar to a diaphragm. Additionally, patients can be taught to remove and replace a ring pessary on their own, giving patients autonomy in deciding when to use and clean the pessary. The ring is available with and without support. The ring with support is used to prevent the cervix from slipping through the ring [55]. The ring pessaries are inserted by folding the pessary in half, and inserting it into the vagina. Once inside the vagina, the pessary is pushed past the cervix into the posterior fornix with the distal edge behind the pubic symphysis. A study by Wu et al. offers a simplified protocol for pessary management where patients were offered a ring pessary either with or without support. Seventy percent of women had successful pessary fittings with a ring pessary [56].

For advanced prolapse, space occupying devices can be used, such as the Gellhorn, donut, or cube pessary [57]. It is important to remember that these shapes are more difficult for patients to self-remove and replace, and may prohibit sexual intercourse. Additionally, these devices can also be associated with greater vaginal discharge and irritation. In patients with SUI, a pessary with a knob may be the preferred option to treat both prolapse and SUI.

Regardless of pessary type chosen, ensuring the correct fit of a pessary is important. When placing a pessary, you should be able to place a finger between pessary and vaginal wall to ensure no undue pressure on the vaginal sidewall. When fitted properly, the patient should not be aware of the pessary and should be able to sit, walk, and void in office without issues. Risk factors for an unsuccessful pessary fit are short vaginal length, large genital hiatus, prior hysterectomy, and prior surgical repair of POP [58–60]. While these can be hurdles for proper fitting, they are not contraindications to fitting a pessary. It is important to discuss with the patient that pessary fitting may take multiple attempts and pessary size required may change over time. If the pessary is expelled while at home, it is appropriate to return to the office for another fitting. As mentioned previously, providers can teach a patient to remove and clean certain devices such as ring and anti-incontinence ring pessaries. This increases patient autonomy and ultimately satisfaction.

It is important to emphasize the need for follow up as this decreases incidence of pessary complications [61]. There is a lack of consensus regarding pessary follow up timeline [52]. A study by Wu et al. offers a simplified protocol for pessary management with follow up every 3 months for the first year and 6 months thereafter,

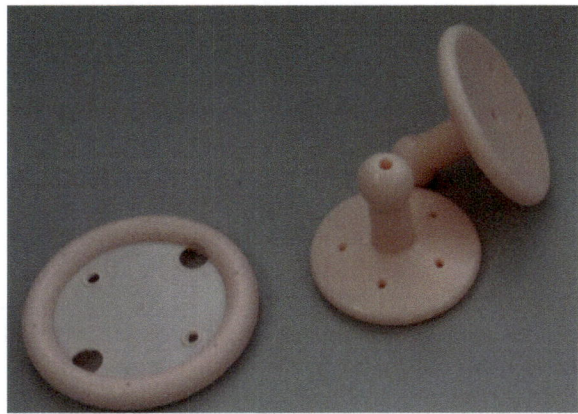

**Fig. 9.6** Ring pessary with support and Gellhorn pessary. (Info: *Huckfinne—Own work, PD-self,* https://commons.wikimedia.org/wiki/File:Pessaries.JPG)

with self-care of the pessary encouraged (Fig. 9.7). There were no serious complications in the study sample of 81 women [56]. This demonstrates the safety of initial follow up of 3 months and suggests that in patients who remove and clean their pessary on their own, follow up can be arranged every 6 months after first year, with no increase in adverse events. Follow-up timelines should be created on a case by case basis to mitigate risk of erosion and serious pessary side effects.

During follow-up visits, patients should be asked about vaginal discharge, bleeding, and difficulty emptying their bowel and bladder. Bacterial vaginosis can occur in up to 30% of patients with a pessary and is less common when removed frequently [62]. Any patient with vaginal bleeding with no ulceration or evidence of vaginal trauma, may require work up for abnormal uterine bleeding. Constipation should be treated with a bowel regimen. A thorough vaginal exam should be performed, where the vaginal epithelium is checked for erosions. For any vaginal erosions identified, consider a period of time without the pessary (up to 2–3 weeks) and vaginal estrogen cream until the erosion is healed. If the vaginal erosion is not healing properly consider biopsy. Persistent vaginal bleeding, even in the presence of vaginal erosions, should prompt an evaluation for an intrauterine source (with transvaginal ultrasound or endometrial biopsy) in women who still have a uterus.

In terms of long-term use, 70–92% of patients using a pessary are satisfied [63, 64] and 50–80% continue at 1 year [58, 65]. However, as time goes on this number decreases with 14–48% of patients maintaining pessary use at 5 years [58]. The reasons for this are various and include pessary fit failure, undesirable side effects and patient preference for a more permanent solution.

## Surgical Management

There are many different surgical techniques for repairing pelvic organ prolapse. The description of the below techniques is meant to give a general guide but is not all-inclusive. The repair of pelvic organ prolapse is broken up into two major categories: obliterative and functional repairs. You can contact your hospital's Obstetrics and Gynecology and Urology departments to find out whether there are physicians board certified in urogynecology (also called Female Pelvic Medicine and Reconstructive Surgery) in your hospital system. You can also visit the American Urogynecologic Society website and use their provider search function.

## Obliterative Repairs

Obliterative repairs offer the most effective repair for POP with success rates ranging from 90 to 100% [66–69]. They can be offered with (total colpocleisis) or without hysterectomy (Le Fort colpocleisis) [70]. Patients should be counseled that they will be unable to have penetrative intercourse if they choose an obliterative repair. Despite this important consideration, in appropriate patients this is an excellent procedure as studies have shown after colpocleisis regret is low [71, 72].

**Fig. 9.7** A simplified protocol for pessary management [56]

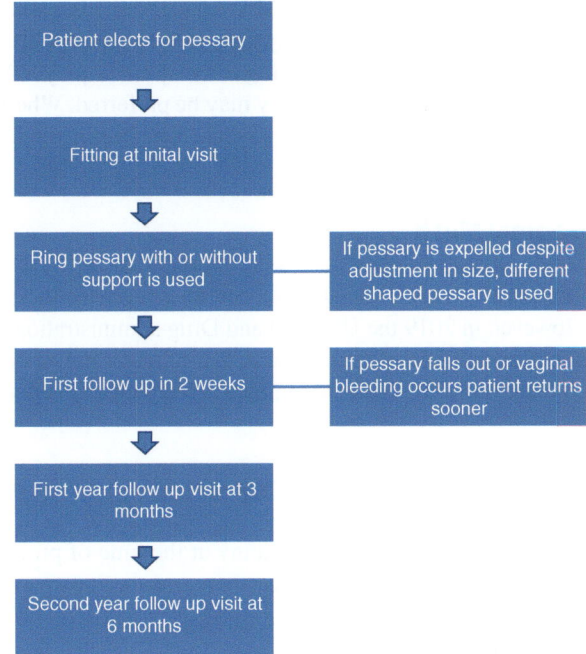

## Functional Repairs

Functional repairs maintain the function of the vagina. There are two main approaches to functional repair of POP: a vaginal approach and an abdominal approach. The vaginal approach to functional repair of POP involves repairing the prolapse using a patient's own native tissue, through the vagina. Sutures are used to suspend the prolapse to various ligaments in the pelvis. In these types of repairs, all incisions are vaginal. In a large study looking at the success of the vaginal approach to functional repair of prolapse, 40% of women had recurrent bothersome prolapse symptoms at 5 years, with approximately 10% undergoing retreatment at 5 years [73].

Sacrocolpopexy is the most common way to repair prolapse abdominally, while still maintaining function of the vagina. A sacrocolpopexy uses surgical mesh to suspend the anterior, posterior, and apical vaginal walls to the anterior longitudinal ligament that runs along the sacrum [74]. This procedure may be done with concomitant hysterectomy, and may be approached via laparotomy or minimally invasive (laparoscopic or robotic) techniques. Laparoscopic and robotic approaches are less invasive, have less blood loss, less post-operative pain, shorter length of stay with no difference in functional or anatomic outcome [75–77].

In terms of efficacy, a systematic review of studies from 1966 to 2004 showed that the success rate for sacrocolpopexy ranged from 76 to 100% with a reoperation rate of approximately 4% up to 3 years [78]. In a study looking at longer term outcomes at 5 years, the surgical success rate was 89% and there were no failures in the apical compartment. The 4% of patients requiring reoperation for POP had native tissue repairs of either the anterior or posterior compartments [79]. When comparing the abdominal sacrocolpopexy approach to repair with vaginal native tissue repair, patient centered decision making is a major role player. When anatomic durability is a priority, mesh sacrocolpopexy may be preferred. When minimizing adverse events is a priority, there is no strong evidence supporting one approach [80–82].

## Vaginal Mesh

Historically vaginal mesh has been an option for the repair of prolapse vaginally. However, in 2019 the US Food and Drug administration (FDA) discontinued the distribution and sale of vaginal mesh kits to repair pelvic organ prolapse [83]. Mesh for mid urethral slings and abdominal sacrocolpopexy is not included in these warnings.

## Concomitant Hysterectomy

Most patients opt for hysterectomy at the time of prolapse repair. For patients that desire to maintain their uterus, there are uterine sparing procedures for repair of POP described [84, 85].

## Recurrence

As noted above, no procedure guarantees complete success. Risk factors for recurrent prolapse include: levator ani avulsion, preoperative stage 3–4, and family history of prolapse [86]. Patients may have a recurrence of anatomic prolapse but may be asymptomatic. In a 2009 study, the absence or presence of bulge symptoms correlated with patient's assessment of improvement while anatomic outcomes did not [87]. Because of this, many studies on repair of POP are moving toward composite outcomes focusing on both patient reported outcomes and objective measurements of anatomic success.

> **Case (Continued)**
> Sandy is greatly appreciative of your comprehensive discussion of pelvic organ prolapse. Since she is asymptomatic, she does not feel that she desires treatment at this time. You agree with her and together you discuss a plan to monitor how she is doing at her yearly exam. As she mentioned before, Sandy has recently had some weight gain. You discuss with her that weight loss may improve her prolapse and her hypertension, as well as improve her quality of life. While she elects for observation now, she found very informative your discussion of treatment options. She thinks in the future if she becomes symptomatic, she would like to try a pessary. She is happy to know a non-surgical option for prolapse treatment exists.

## Summary/Conclusion

In conclusion, pelvic organ prolapse (POP) is common among postmenopausal women. For the provider taking care of this population, it is important to take a through history to screen for POP, as well as perform a comprehensive physical exam to assess the extent of POP. It is important for the provider to understand that the treatment of POP consists of both conservative and surgical options. Being able to discuss with patients the conservative management of POP, including observation, physical therapy, and pessary placement is crucial. Furthermore, for the patient who desires surgical management, it is important for providers to be able to help patients navigate surgical options in conjunction with specialists.

## References

1. Abrams P, Cardozo L, Fall M, et al. The standardisation of terminology of lower urinary tract function: report from the Standardisation Sub-committee of the International Continence Society. Neurourol Urodyn. 2002;21(2):167–78.
2. Hendrix SL, Clark A, Nygaard I, et al. Pelvic organ prolapse in the Women's Health Initiative: gravity and gravidity. Am J Obstet Gynecol. 2002;186(6):1160–6.
3. Wu JM, Vaughan CP, Goode PS, et al. Prevalence and trends of symptomatic pelvic floor disorders in U.S. women. Obstet Gynecol. 2014;123(1):141–8.
4. Wu JM, Matthews CA, Conover MM, Pate V, Funk MJ. Lifetime risk of stress incontinence or pelvic organ prolapse surgery. Obstet Gynecol. 2014;123(6):1201.
5. Wu JM, Hundley AF, Fulton RG, Myers ER. Forecasting the prevalence of pelvic floor disorders in U.S. women: 2010 to 2050. Obstet Gynecol. 2009;114(6):1278–83.
6. Sung VW, Washington B, Raker CA. Costs of ambulatory care related to female pelvic floor disorders in the United States. Am J Obstet Gynecol. 2010;202(5):483.e481–4.
7. Vergeldt TF, Weemhoff M, IntHout J, Kluivers KB. Risk factors for pelvic organ prolapse and its recurrence: a systematic review. Int Urogynecol J. 2015;26(11):1559–73.
8. Mothes A, Radosa M, Altendorf-Hofmann A, Runnebaum IB. Risk index for pelvic organ prolapse based on established individual risk factors. Arch Gynecol Obstet. 2016;293(3):617–24.
9. Blomquist JL, Muñoz A, Carroll M, Handa VL. Association of delivery mode with pelvic floor disorders after childbirth. JAMA. 2018;320(23):2438–47.
10. Moalli PA, Ivy SJ, Meyn LA, Zyczynski HM. Risk factors associated with pelvic floor disorders in women undergoing surgical repair. Obstet Gynecol. 2003;101(5):869–74.
11. Handa VL, Blomquist JL, Knoepp LR, et al. Pelvic floor disorders 5-10 years after vaginal or cesarean childbirth. Obstet Gynecol. 2011;118(4):777.
12. Mant J, Painter R, Vessey M. Epidemiology of genital prolapse: observations from the Oxford Family Planning Association Study. BJOG Int J Obstet Gynaecol. 1997;104(5):579–85.
13. Swift S, Woodman P, O'Boyle A, et al. Pelvic Organ Support Study (POSST): the distribution, clinical definition, and epidemiologic condition of pelvic organ support defects. Am J Obstet Gynecol. 2005;192(3):795–806.
14. Luber KM, Boero S, Choe JY. The demographics of pelvic floor disorders: current observations and future projections. Am J Obstet Gynecol. 2001;184(7):1496–501; discussion 1501-1493.
15. Swift SE, Tate SB, Nicholas J. Correlation of symptoms with degree of pelvic organ support in a general population of women: what is pelvic organ prolapse? Am J Obstet Gynecol. 2003;189(2):372–7.
16. Giri A, Hartmann KE, Hellwege JN, Velez Edwards DR, Edwards TL. Obesity and pelvic organ prolapse: a systematic review and meta-analysis of observational studies. Am J Obstet Gynecol. 2017;217(1):11–26.e13.

17. Lian W, Zheng Y, Huang H, Chen L, Cao B. Effects of bariatric surgery on pelvic floor disorders in obese women: a meta-analysis. Arch Gynecol Obstet. 2017;296(2):181–9.
18. Spence-Jones C, Kamm MA, Henry MM, Hudson CN. Bowel dysfunction: a pathogenic factor in uterovaginal prolapse and urinary stress incontinence. BJOG Int J Obstet Gynaecol. 1994;101(2):147–52.
19. Kahn MA, Breitkopf CR, Valley MT, et al. Pelvic Organ Support Study (POSST) and bowel symptoms: straining at stool is associated with perineal and anterior vaginal descent in a general gynecologic population. Am J Obstet Gynecol. 2005;192(5):1516–22.
20. Jelovsek JE, Barber MD, Paraiso MFR, Walters MD. Functional bowel and anorectal disorders in patients with pelvic organ prolapse and incontinence. Am J Obstet Gynecol. 2005;193(6):2105–11.
21. Weber AM, Walters MD, Ballard LA, Booher DL, Piedmonte MR. Posterior vaginal prolapse and bowel function. Am J Obstet Gynecol. 1998;179(6):1446–50.
22. Jørgensen S, Hein H, Gyntelberg F. Heavy lifting at work and risk of genital prolapse and herniated lumbar disc in assistant nurses. Occup Med. 1994;44(1):47–9.
23. DeLancey JO, Kearney R, Chou Q, Speights S, Binno S. The appearance of levator ani muscle abnormalities in magnetic resonance images after vaginal delivery. Obstet Gynecol. 2003;101(1):46–53.
24. Lien K-C, Mooney B, DeLancey JO, Ashton-Miller JA. Levator ani muscle stretch induced by simulated vaginal birth. Obstet Gynecol. 2004;103(1):31.
25. DeLancey JO. The hidden epidemic of pelvic floor dysfunction: achievable goals for improved prevention and treatment. Am J Obstet Gynecol. 2005;192(5):1488–95.
26. Carley ME, Schaffer J. Urinary incontinence and pelvic organ prolapse in women with Marfan or Ehlers-Danlos syndrome. Am J Obstet Gynecol. 2000;182(5):1021–3.
27. Jelovsek JE, Barber MD. Women seeking treatment for advanced pelvic organ prolapse have decreased body image and quality of life. Am J Obstet Gynecol. 2006;194(5):1455–61.
28. Handa VL, Cundiff G, Chang HH, Helzlsouer KJ. Female sexual function and pelvic floor disorders. Obstet Gynecol. 2008;111(5):1045.
29. Lowder JL, Ghetti C, Nikolajski C, Oliphant SS, Zyczynski HM. Body image perceptions in women with pelvic organ prolapse: a qualitative study. Am J Obstet Gynecol. 2011;204(5):441.e441–5.
30. Barber MD, Neubauer NL, Klein-Olarte V. Can we screen for pelvic organ prolapse without a physical examination in epidemiologic studies? Am J Obstet Gynecol. 2006;195(4):942–8.
31. Lawrence JM, Lukacz ES, Nager CW, Hsu J-WY, Luber KM. Prevalence and co-occurrence of pelvic floor disorders in community-dwelling women. Obstet Gynecol. 2008;111(3):678–85.
32. DeLancey JO. Fascial and muscular abnormalities in women with urethral hypermobility and anterior vaginal wall prolapse. Am J Obstet Gynecol. 2002;187(1):93–8.
33. DeLancey JO. Structural support of the urethra as it relates to stress urinary incontinence: the hammock hypothesis. Am J Obstet Gynecol. 1994;170(5):1713–23.
34. Coates K, Harris R, Cundiff G, Bump RC. Uroflowmetry in women with urinary incontinence and pelvic organ prolapse. Br J Urol. 1997;80(2):217–21.
35. Kenton K, Shott S, Brubaker L. Vaginal topography does not correlate well with visceral position in women with pelvic organ prolapse. Int Urogynecol J Pelvic Floor Dysfunct. 1997;8(6):336–9.
36. Bump RC, Mattiasson A, Bø K, et al. The standardization of terminology of female pelvic organ prolapse and pelvic floor dysfunction. Am J Obstet Gynecol. 1996;175(1):10–7.
37. Brubaker L, Carberry C, Nardos R, Carter-Brooks C, Lowder JL. American Urogynecologic Society best practice statement: evaluation and counseling of patients with pelvic organ prolapse. Female Pelvic Med Reconstr Surg. 2017;23(5):281–7.
38. Toozs-Hobson P, Freeman R, Barber M, et al. An International Urogynecological Association (IUGA)/International Continence Society (ICS) joint report on the terminology for reporting outcomes of surgical procedures for pelvic organ prolapse. Int Urogynecol J. 2012;23(5):527–35.

39. Percy JP, Neill ME, Swash M, Parks AG. Electrophysiological study of motor nerve supply of pelvic floor. Lancet (London, England). 1981;1(8210):16–7.
40. Weber AM, Richter HE. Pelvic organ prolapse. Obstet Gynecol. 2005;106(3):615–34.
41. Hagen S, Stark D, Glazener C, et al. Individualised pelvic floor muscle training in women with pelvic organ prolapse (POPPY): a multicentre randomised controlled trial. Lancet. 2014;383(9919):796–806.
42. Wiegersma M, Panman CM, Kollen BJ, Berger MY, Lisman-Van Leeuwen Y, Dekker JH. Effect of pelvic floor muscle training compared with watchful waiting in older women with symptomatic mild pelvic organ prolapse: randomised controlled trial in primary care. BMJ. 2014;349:g7378.
43. Piya-Anant M, Therasakvichya S, Leelaphatanadit C, Techatrisak K. Integrated health research program for the Thai elderly: prevalence of genital prolapse and effectiveness of pelvic floor exercise to prevent worsening of genital prolapse in elderly women. J Med Assoc Thail. 2003;86(6):509–15.
44. Cundiff GW, Amundsen CL, Bent AE, et al. The PESSRI study: symptom relief outcomes of a randomized crossover trial of the ring and Gellhorn pessaries. Am J Obstet Gynecol. 2007;196(4):405.e401–8.
45. Abdool Z, Thakar R, Sultan AH, Oliver RS. Prospective evaluation of outcome of vaginal pessaries versus surgery in women with symptomatic pelvic organ prolapse. Int Urogynecol J. 2011;22(3):273–8.
46. Barber MD, Walters MD, Cundiff GW. Responsiveness of the Pelvic Floor Distress Inventory (PFDI) and Pelvic Floor Impact Questionnaire (PFIQ) in women undergoing vaginal surgery and pessary treatment for pelvic organ prolapse. Am J Obstet Gynecol. 2006;194(5):1492–8.
47. Fernando RJ, Thakar R, Sultan AH, Shah SM, Jones PW. Effect of vaginal pessaries on symptoms associated with pelvic organ prolapse. Obstet Gynecol. 2006;108(1):93–9.
48. Jones K, Yang L, Lowder JL, et al. Effect of pessary use on genital hiatus measurements in women with pelvic organ prolapse. Obstet Gynecol. 2008;112(3):630–6.
49. Komesu YM, Rogers RG, Rode MA, et al. Pelvic floor symptom changes in pessary users. Am J Obstet Gynecol. 2007;197(6):620.e621–6.
50. Kuhn A, Bapst D, Stadlmayr W, Vits K, Mueller MD. Sexual and organ function in patients with symptomatic prolapse: are pessaries helpful? Fertil Steril. 2009;91(5):1914–8.
51. Patel M, Mellen C, O'Sullivan DM, LaSala CA. Impact of pessary use on prolapse symptoms, quality of life, and body image. Am J Obstet Gynecol. 2010;202(5):499.e491–4.
52. Cundiff GW, Weidner AC, Visco AG, Bump RC, Addison WA. A survey of pessary use by members of the American Urogynecologic Society. Obstet Gynecol. 2000;95(6 Pt 1):931–5.
53. Obstetricians ACOG. Pelvic organ prolapse. ACOG practice bulletin number 176. Obstet Gynecol. 2017;129:56–72.
54. Pott-Grinstein E, Newcomer JR. Gynecologists' patterns of prescribing pessaries. J Reprod Med. 2001;46(3):205–8.
55. Trowbridge ER, Fenner DE. Conservative management of pelvic organ prolapse. Clin Obstet Gynecol. 2005;48(3):668–81.
56. Wu V, Farrell SA, Baskett TF, Flowerdew G. A simplified protocol for pessary management. Obstet Gynecol. 1997;90(6):990–4.
57. Clemons JL, Aguilar VC, Tillinghast TA, Jackson ND, Myers DL. Risk factors associated with an unsuccessful pessary fitting trial in women with pelvic organ prolapse. Am J Obstet Gynecol. 2004;190(2):345–50.
58. Lamers BH, Broekman BM, Milani AL. Pessary treatment for pelvic organ prolapse and health-related quality of life: a review. Int Urogynecol J. 2011;22(6):637.
59. Maito JM, Quam ZA, Craig E, Dannerq KA, Rogers RG. Predictors of successful pessary fitting and continued use in a nurse-midwifery pessary clinic. J Midwifery Women's Health. 2006;51(2):78–84.
60. Mutone MF, Terry C, Hale DS, Benson JT. Factors which influence the short-term success of pessary management of pelvic organ prolapse. Am J Obstet Gynecol. 2005;193(1):89–94.

61. Arias BE, Ridgeway B, Barber MD. Complications of neglected vaginal pessaries: case presentation and literature review. Int Urogynecol J Pelvic Floor Dysfunct. 2008;19(8):1173–8.
62. Meriwether KV, Rogers RG, Craig E, et al. The effect of hydroxyquinoline-based gel on pessary-associated bacterial vaginosis: a multicenter randomized controlled trial. Am J Obstet Gynecol. 2015;213(5):729.e721–9.
63. Bai SW, Yoon BS, Kwon JY, Shin JS, Kim SK, Park KH. Survey of the characteristics and satisfaction degree of the patients using a pessary. Int Urogynecol J. 2005;16(3):182–6.
64. Clemons JL, Aguilar VC, Tillinghast TA, Jackson ND, Myers DL. Patient satisfaction and changes in prolapse and urinary symptoms in women who were fitted successfully with a pessary for pelvic organ prolapse. Am J Obstet Gynecol. 2004;190(4):1025–9.
65. Clemons JL, Aguilar VC, Sokol ER, Jackson ND, Myers DL. Patient characteristics that are associated with continued pessary use versus surgery after 1 year. Am J Obstet Gynecol. 2004;191(1):159–64.
66. Fitzgerald MP, Richter HE, Bradley CS, et al. Pelvic support, pelvic symptoms, and patient satisfaction after colpocleisis. Int Urogynecol J Pelvic Floor Dysfunct. 2008;19(12):1603–9.
67. DeLancey JO, Morley GW. Total colpocleisis for vaginal eversion. Am J Obstet Gynecol. 1997;176(6):1228–32; discussion 1232-1225.
68. FitzGerald MP, Brubaker L. Colpocleisis and urinary incontinence. Am J Obstet Gynecol. 2003;189(5):1241–4.
69. Misrai V, Gosseine PN, Costa P, Haab F, Delmas V. Colpocleisis: indications, technique and results. Prog Urol. 2009;19(13):1031–6.
70. Hoffman MS, Cardosi RJ, Lockhart J, Hall DC, Murphy SJ. Vaginectomy with pelvic herniorrhaphy for prolapse. Am J Obstet Gynecol. 2003;189(2):364–70; discussion 370-361.
71. Crisp CC, Book NM, Cunkelman JA, Tieu AL, Pauls RN. Body image, regret, and satisfaction 24 weeks after colpocleisis: a multicenter study. Female Pelvic Med Reconstr Surg. 2016;22(3):132–5.
72. Wang X, Chen Y, Hua K. Pelvic symptoms, body image, and regret after LeFort colpocleisis: a long-term follow-up. J Minim Invasive Gynecol. 2017;24(3):415–9.
73. Barber MD, Brubaker L, Burgio KL, et al. Comparison of 2 transvaginal surgical approaches and perioperative behavioral therapy for apical vaginal prolapse: the OPTIMAL randomized trial. JAMA. 2014;311(10):1023–34.
74. Schachar JS, Matthews CA. Robotic-assisted repair of pelvic organ prolapse: a scoping review of the literature. Transl Androl Urol. 2019;9:959–70.
75. Geller EJ, Siddiqui NY, Wu JM, Visco AG. Short-term outcomes of robotic sacrocolpopexy compared with abdominal sacrocolpopexy. Obstet Gynecol. 2008;112(6):1201–6.
76. Coolen AWM, van Oudheusden AMJ, Mol BWJ, van Eijndhoven HWF, Roovers JWR, Bongers MY. Laparoscopic sacrocolpopexy compared with open abdominal sacrocolpopexy for vault prolapse repair: a randomised controlled trial. Int Urogynecol J. 2017;28(10):1469–79.
77. Paraiso MF, Walters MD, Rackley RR, Melek S, Hugney C. Laparoscopic and abdominal sacral colpopexies: a comparative cohort study. Am J Obstet Gynecol. 2005;192(5):1752–8.
78. Nygaard IE, McCreery R, Brubaker L, et al. Abdominal sacrocolpopexy: a comprehensive review. Obstet Gynecol. 2004;104(4):805–23.
79. Culligan PJ, Lewis C, Priestley J, Mushonga N. Long-term outcomes of robotic-assisted laparoscopic sacrocolpopexy using lightweight Y-mesh. Female Pelvic Med Reconstr Surg. 2019;26:202–6.
80. Siddiqui NY, Grimes CL, Casiano ER, et al. Mesh sacrocolpopexy compared with native tissue vaginal repair: a systematic review and meta-analysis. Obstet Gynecol. 2015;125(1):44.
81. Benson JT, Lucente V, McClellan E. Vaginal versus abdominal reconstructive surgery for the treatment of pelvic support defects: a prospective randomized study with long-term outcome evaluation. Am J Obstet Gynecol. 1996;175(6):1418–22.
82. Maher C, Feiner B, Baessler K, Schmid C. Surgical management of pelvic organ prolapse in women. Cochrane Database Syst Rev. 2013;4:CD004014.

83. Administration FaD. Urogynecologic Surgical Mesh Implants. https://www.fda.gov/medical-devices/implants-and-prosthetics/urogynecologic-surgical-mesh-implants. Published 2019 Accessed 19 June 2019.
84. Bovbjerg VE, Trowbridge ER, Barber MD, et al. Patient-centered treatment goals for pelvic floor disorders: association with quality-of-life and patient satisfaction. Am J Obstet Gynecol. 2009;200(5):568.e561–6.
85. Pakbaz M, Persson M, Löfgren M, Mogren I. 'A hidden disorder until the pieces fall into place'-a qualitative study of vaginal prolapse. BMC Womens Health. 2010;10(1):18.
86. Friedman T, Eslick GD, Dietz HP. Risk factors for prolapse recurrence: systematic review and meta-analysis. Int Urogynecol J. 2018;29(1):13–21.
87. Barber MD, Brubaker L, Nygaard I, Wheeler TL. Defining success after surgery for pelvic organ prolapse. Obstet Gynecol. 2009;114(3):600.

# Vulvar Pathology in Older Women

**10**

Emily R. Rosen

---

**Key Points**
1. Nearly half of all postmenopausal women will experience vulvovaginal complaints.
2. There are common physiologic changes in postmenopausal patients that increase the likelihood of vulvar pathology.
3. Possible etiologies for vulvovaginal complaints include dermatitis, atrophy, infection, vulvar dermatosis, malignancy, and manifestations of other chronic diseases.
4. Any lesion that appears abnormal, does not improve with treatment, or occurs in a high-risk patient should be biopsied.
5. Though cure may not be possible, a long-term patient-provider partnership is necessary for vulvar symptom management and surveillance.

---

**Case**
Edith is a 71-year-old patient who presents to your office reporting vulvar itching. The itching started approximately 2 years ago, but she thought her symptoms were "due to aging." However, the itching has become more persistent and bothersome over the past 3 months. She reports that her symptoms are worse at the end of the day. You take a history and determine that Edith has a diagnosis of hypertension, stress urinary incontinence, and depression. Her medications include lisinopril, venlafaxine, a multivitamin, vitamin D, and evening primrose oil.

---

E. R. Rosen (✉)
Department of Obstetrics and Gynecology, The Ohio State University, Columbus, OH, USA
e-mail: Emily.rosen@osumc.edu

## How to Begin a Conversation Regarding Vulvar Complaints

It is important to provide reassurance and support when a patient presents with vulvovaginal symptoms. Many women do not disclose their concerns due to embarrassment, fear, and the false belief that vulvar symptoms are normal in older women. However, vulvar symptoms are common in postmenopausal women and often require treatment. Patients should be informed that symptoms are common and that relief is possible [1, 2]. Although symptom improvement is achievable, treatment often requires several office visits, possible biopsies, various treatment attempts, and potential referral to other specialists.

## Common Vulvar Symptoms

Common vulvar complaints include pruritus, burning, pain, dyspareunia, discharge, bleeding, or a new lesion. Symptoms can be acute or chronic. Since most vulvar symptoms are not specific to a particular vulvar condition, elucidating the diagnosis can be challenging.

## Important Questions to Ask Edith Before the Exam

The initial evaluation should include a detailed symptom characterization and past medical history focusing on chronic medical conditions, current medications, sexual history, and vulvar hygiene practices. Essential elements of the history can be found in Table 10.1.

**Table 10.1** Initial history in a patient with vulvar complaints

| Symptom characterization | Past medical history | Other focused questions |
|---|---|---|
| Onset | Chronic medical issues | Vulvar hygiene practices |
| Duration |   History of autoimmune disorders |   Excessive washing |
| Location |   Dermatologic history |   Use of scented body soaps |
| Frequency and severity | Obstetric and gynecologic history |   Laundry products |
| Precipitating factors |   History of vulvar disorders | Sexual practices |
| Relieving factors |   History of pelvic infections | Occlusive clothing |
| Attempted treatments |   History of abnormal pap smears | Application of medications/agents to the vulva |
| |   Vaginal bleeding | Impact of symptoms on quality of life |
| |   Incontinence | |
| | Immunocompromised status | |
| | Medications | |

It is imperative to review the urogenital anatomy and clarify the location of a patient's symptoms as many women report "vaginal" symptoms when they actually intend to refer to vulvar concerns.

> **Best Practice**
> Do not forget to obtain a thorough medical history! Systemic diseases, such as Crohn disease or psoriasis, can have vulvar manifestations.

> **Case (Continued)**
> Edith reports that she has been using topical antibacterial ointment that she purchased over the counter. Despite this, she continues to have symptoms.

## Causes of Vulvar Symptoms

Many vulvar irritants are routinely used in our daily lives and vulvar hygiene practices. These include prescription and nonprescription therapies that can precipitate the itch-scratch cycle that is commonly reported in patients with vulvar symptoms. Table 10.2 provides a list of common irritants and allergens. Patients should be asked whether they are using any of these irritants to guide appropriate counseling.

The hormonal changes associated with menopause result in physiologic and anatomic changes of the vulva and vagina. The hypoestrogenic state of menopause

**Table 10.2** Common vulvar irritants [3]

| |
|---|
| Adult or baby wipes |
| Antiseptic solutions |
| Bathroom products—soaps, shampoo, conditioner, bath salts, scented toilet paper |
| Body fluid—semen, saliva, sweat, urine |
| Contraceptive creams, lubricants, and latex |
| Dyes |
| Hygiene products—deodorants, perfumes, sprays, powders |
| Laundry products—detergents, fabric softeners, dryer sheets |
| Sanity products—pads, tampons |
| Topical products—creams, ointments, moisturizers, anesthetics (lidocaine, benzocaine), antibacterial, and antimycotics |
| Topical steroids |
| Topical medications—trichloroacetic acid, 5-fluorouracil, podofilox, or podophyllin |

results in an increased vaginal pH, reduced vaginal blood flow, and decreased vaginal secretions. These changes, in the setting of impaired cell-medicated immunity and tissue regeneration capacity, result in decreased antimicrobial defenses and an increased risk of urogenital infections. Patients may also experience vulvovaginal discomfort, dyspareunia (pain with intercourse), and urinary symptoms. These physiologic changes are collectively referred to as genitourinary syndrome of menopause (GSM). More information about this condition can be found in Chapter 1.

A nice graphic depicting vulvar and vaginal changes related to menopause can be found here [4]. Due to these changes, the vulva becomes more vulnerable to mechanical trauma and chemical irritation. Additionally, the increased prevalence of urinary and fecal incontinence in postmenopausal women can exacerbate vulvar symptoms.

The combination of estrogen deficiency, impaired immunity, increased susceptibility to mechanical and chemical injury, and prevalence of skin disorders in postmenopausal women place them at a significantly increased risk of vulvar pathology [5–7].

## How to Perform a Complete Vulvovaginal Exam

When performing an exam, providers should:
1. Assess for signs of vulvar and vaginal atrophy (GSM)
2. Look for evidence of infection and perform specific testing if needed
3. Evaluate areas of vulvar hypo-/hyperpigmentation, new lesions, vascularity, or evidence of trauma, noting whether changes are focal or generalized
4. Consider a global skin exam, including the oral mucosa, to help narrow the differential

Common postmenopausal vulvar changes may include loss of labial fat pads, sparse pubic hair, and atrophy that can result in excoriations, agglutination, and loss of normal vulvar architecture. Common vaginal changes in older women include loss of vaginal rugae, mucosal pallor, vaginal dryness, and decreased vaginal length and diameter [4, 8].

## What Types of Infections Can Cause Vaginitis?

Although Edith's exam does not reveal any signs of infection, infections are a common cause of vaginal and vulvar complaints. Therefore, it is prudent to test for infectious etiologies when a woman, regardless of her age, presents with vaginitis.

The most common causes of infectious vaginitis are candidiasis, bacterial vaginosis, and trichomonas. The majority of women will be diagnosed with a vaginal infection during their lifetime. Diagnosis of vaginitis includes a combination of patient symptoms, vulvovaginal exam, vaginal fluid pH and microscopy, and other tests if needed (see Table 10.3). To perform a vaginal pH test, press a pH paper strip to the upper vaginal wall for a few seconds and then match the pH strip color to the

Table 10.3 Overview of causes, symptoms, and diagnosis of infectious vaginitis [10, 11]

| Infection | Cause | Physical exam | Testing | Symptoms | Risk factors and fun facts | Treatment |
|---|---|---|---|---|---|---|
| Vulvovaginal candidiasis | Candida species: *Candida albicans* > *C. tropicalis*, *C. glabrata* | Vulvar inflammation and erythema, thick white discharge | pH: Normal (<4.5) Saline wet mount: yeast buds and pseudohyphae KOH prep: Pseudohyphae and budding yeast Others: Yeast culture, Affirm | Thick white often curdy discharge, pruritus, edema, dyspareunia, dysuria, odorless | Immunosuppression, HIV, steroid use, recent antibiotic use, uncontrolled diabetes | Over-the-counter intravaginal, prescription intravaginal, and oral agents are available Fluconazole 150 mg orally once is the most common regimen Additional treatment regimens can be found in [11] |
| Bacterial vaginosis | Anaerobic bacteria (prevotella, mobiluncus, gardnerella vaginalis, ureaplasma, mycoplasma) | No vulvar inflammation, thin, watery, white-gray discharge, fishy odor | pH: ↑ (>4.5) Saline wet mount: Clue cells (>20%) KOH prep: + whiff test Others: Amsel criteria [10]; Gram stain with Nugent scoring; Affirm | Thin, watery, white-gray discharge, fishy odor | Low SES, smoking, multiple sexual partners, vaginal douching, women who have sex with women *Note*: BV increases risk of post-surgical infections and HIV transmission | Metronidazole: 500 mg orally BID for 7 days *or* 0.75% gel 5 gram (1 full applicator) intravaginally daily for 5 days Clindamycin cream 2%: 5 gram (1 full applicator) intravaginally qhs for 7 days See [11] for alternative treatment options |
| Trichomonas | Trichomonas vaginalis | Classic discharge, vaginal and cervical erythema, strawberry cervix | pH: ↑ (>4.5) Saline wet mount: Motile trichomonads, many PMNs KOH prep: Variable whiff test Others: NAAT, Affirm, culture | Yellow-green frothy discharge, pruritus, vaginal soreness, dysuria, odor | Low SES, multiple sexual partners, presence of other STIs *Note*: For information on expedited partner therapy in your state, see https://www.cdc.gov/std/ept/legal/default.htm Make sure to screen for other STIs! | Metronidazole 500 mg orally BID for 7 days *or* 2 grams orally once Alternative treatment option: tinidazole 2 grams orally once Simultaneous expedited partner therapy (EPT) is key to treatment! |

color chart on the pH strip dispenser. For more information on how to perform and analyze a wet mount, watch this brief video: https://www.youtube.com/watch?v=8dgeOPGx6YI [9].

Symptom resolution occurs with appropriate treatment; however, infections can recur and be more complicated. For information on recurrent or complicated vaginitis treatment, consult additional references (10, 11).

- Nearly all providers will encounter vulvovaginal candidiasis. Up to 75% of women will be diagnosed with vulvovaginal candidiasis in their lifetime, and 40–45% of patients will have more than one infection [12]. Vulvovaginal candidiasis is classified as complicated on uncomplicated based upon the frequency of infections, species of candida and other patient factors. Topical or oral antifungals are appropriate treatment options, depending on the classification of the infection.
  - Uncomplicated: mild–moderate disease, <4 infections/year, *Candida albicans*
  - Complicated: moderate–severe disease, >4 infections/year, non-*Candida albicans*, adverse host factors (immunocompromised, diabetes, etc.) [10]
- Bacterial vaginosis occurs when the normal vaginal flora shifts and an overgrowth of anaerobic bacteria replace lactobacillus species.
- Trichomonas is a sexually transmitted infection that causes increased discharge and dyspareunia, but rarely results in pruritus.

> **Best Practice**
> There has been a consistent rise in the prevalence of STIs in postmenopausal women over the past decade! [13] This may be due to the false belief that they are at lower risk for contracting STIs, high divorce rate, and more outlets for social networking. It is important to discuss sexual history with all patients and screen for STIs when indicated. Perform a yeast culture if wet mounts are persistently positive or if a patient is unresponsive to treatment!

> **Case (Continued)**
> After the exam, you inform Edith that she has GSM and contact dermatitis. You tell her that GSM is very common in post-menopausal women and is due to decreased estrogen. You provide handouts about vulvar health and hygiene and counsel her about lifestyle modifications and medication options.

The American College of Obstetricians and Gynecologists (ACOG) has excellent patient information on its website.

- Vaginitis: https://www.acog.org/patient-resources/faqs/gynecologic-problems/vaginitis
- Vulvovaginal Health (including GSM): https://www.acog.org/patient-resources/faqs/womens-health/vulvovaginal-health

## How Do You Treat Genitourinary Syndrome of Menopause (GSM)?

A comprehensive overview of the treatment of GSM can be found in Chapter 1 of this book. Treatment options include lifestyle modifications, vaginal lubricants and moisturizers, stimulatory activities to increase vaginal blood flow, and hormonal treatments (See also Chapter 1).
- Lifestyle modifications
  - Encourage smoking cessation. Tobacco use may alter estrogen metabolism and result in increased rates of vaginal atrophy [4].
  - Avoid common allergens and irritants (see Table 10.2).
- Lubricants
- Moisturizers
- Stimulatory activities to increase vaginal blood flow [4, 14]
  - Painless sexual activity (including masturbation)
  - Vaginal dilators
- Hormonal options (vaginal estrogen)

## How Do You Treat Contact Dermatitis? [15]

Contact dermatitis is inflammation or a rash of the skin due to an irritant or allergen. The dermatitis can occur on any area that is exposed to an offending agent, and can have an acute or insidious onset. Patients often report itching, burning, and vulvar irritation. The clinical appearance varies from mild to marked erythema and swelling to ulcers, scaling, vesicles, and evidence of lichenification or altered pigmentation in chronic cases [16]. The skin changes are in the distribution of the contact with the offending agent.

The fundamental treatment strategies for contact dermatitis include the following:
1. Modification of clothing or hygiene habits that promote dermatitis. See "DOs and DO NOTs" for suggested alternative habits.
2. Avoidance of known or suspected environmental irritants (refer to Table 10.2).
3. Exclude underlying diagnoses that may lead to contact dermatitis.
4. Consider topical steroid treatment, the usual treatment of choice.

The International Society for the Study of Vulvovaginal Disease has a patient information sheet about contact dermatitis: https://3b64we1rtwev2ibv6q12s4dd-wpengine.netdna-ssl.com/wp-content/uploads/2016/03/ContactDermatitis-2013-final.pdf [17].

The "DOs and DO NOTs" of Vulvar Hygiene [18, 19]
- DO NOT wear tight clothing (pantyhose, tight pants such as exercise pants, swimsuits, leotards, thongs). DO wear loose pants, skirts, or dresses.
- DO NOT wear synthetic underwear or clothing. DO wear cotton.
- DO NOT use scented soaps, shampoos, or conditioners. DO use fragrance-free pH neutral soap (e.g., Cetaphil, Neutrogena, and pure olive oil soap).
- DO NOT use a bubble bath. DO bathe without additives.
- DO NOT use scented detergents. DO use unscented detergents.
- DO NOT use feminine sprays, douches, or powders. DO inform patients that these products are unnecessary.
- DO NOT use dyed toilet articles. DO use toilet articles without dyes.
- DO NOT use panty liners. DO use cotton pads.
- DO NOT use baby wipes. DO rinse with water.
- DO NOT use washcloths. DO use fingertips for washing and pat dry.

> **Case (Continued)**
>
> Through shared decision making, Edith decides to proceed with lifestyle interventions only. At her 3-month follow-up appointment, she continues to report vulvar itching, burning, and dyspareunia and is prescribed local vaginal estrogen cream. At her next visit, she reports significant improvement.
>
> Edith's friend Carol presents to clinic reporting similar symptoms of vulvar pruritus. Carol knows how happy Edith was with her treatment and is hoping that you can help her, too. Carol is 79 years old and reports vulvar itching and burning. She tried to examine her vulva and noticed some "white coloring on the outside." Edith reports a history of hypothyroidism, but is otherwise healthy.

## What Is Lichen Sclerosis and What Else Might This Be?
(Refer to Table 10.4)

Lichen sclerosis is a common chronic vulvar skin disorder, but its true incidence is unknown since many patients are asymptomatic. The etiology of lichen sclerosis is most likely multifactorial with a possible autoimmune and genetic link. Up to 60% of patients with lichen sclerosis have an autoimmune disorder including vitiligo, alopecia, thyroid disease, and pernicious anemia [20, 21]. Patients typically present with pruritus, but may also report burning and dyspareunia, or may be asymptomatic.

Clinical manifestations are most commonly seen in the anogenital area; however, 11% of women will have extragenital lesions (neck, shoulder, and breasts) [20]. Vaginal involvement has not been documented. The most common description of lichen sclerosis is thinned, whitened skin classically identified as "cigarette paper" that often presents in a figure-of eight, or hourglass, pattern around the vulva and

**Table 10.4** Common vulvar dermatoses

|  | Symptoms | Exam findings | Histopathology | Treatment |
|---|---|---|---|---|
| Lichen sclerosis | Often asymptomatic. Most common symptom is pruritus, but also presents with burning and dyspareunia | Thinned, atrophic, whitened skin with a "cigarette paper" appearance. Classic hourglass pattern around the vulva and anus. Loss of architecture due to agglutination | Epidermal atrophy with loss of rete pegs, upper dermis collagen homogenization with a band-like infiltrate, and hyperkeratosis | Ultra-high potency topical steroid—most commonly clobetasol propionate 0.05% |
| Lichen simplex chronicus | Intense itching that is worse at night | Varies from exaggerated skin lines and broken pubic hair to lichenified skin with altered pigmentation, ulcers, and erosions | Elongation and thickening of rete pegs, thickening of the epidermis | Removal of the offending agent ± low potency topical steroids |
| Lichen planus | Pain, burning, postcoital bleeding | Genital lesions range from pink ill-defined lesions to erosive lesions that cause heavy vaginal discharge and significant loss of architecture. Skin lesions are flat-topped papules and plaques. Wickham striae on papules and on oral mucosa | Band-like lymphocytic infiltrate in the dermo-epidermal junction | High potency topical steroid |

anus. Other common findings include fusion or loss of labia minora, phimosis of the clitoral hood, narrowing of the vaginal introitus, interlabial sulci and posterior fourchette fissures, and ulcers (Fig. 10.1).

There is no cure for lichen sclerosis, but treatment results in disease stabilization. In addition to providing symptom relief, treatment is essential to prevent anatomic changes and possibly prevent malignant transformation [20]. A biopsy should be performed to confirm the diagnosis.

A 1.5 min video about how to perform a vulvar punch biopsy can be found here: https://www.youtube.com/watch?v=T3G6RapA7gA [22]. Histopathology of lichen sclerosis has specific features including loss of rete pegs, upper dermis collagen homogenization with a band-like inflammatory infiltrate, and hyperkeratosis.

If disease does not stabilize with treatment, consider repeat biopsy and/or referral to a gynecologist or vulvar dermatologist.

Although no specific steroid regimen has been shown to be superior, a taper of an ultra-potent topical corticosteroid, most commonly clobetasol propionate 0.05%, is the treatment of choice. Using a mirror, the patient should be instructed where to apply the ointment. The ointment should be applied in a very thin layer, as heavier application may result in exacerbation of vulvar symptoms.

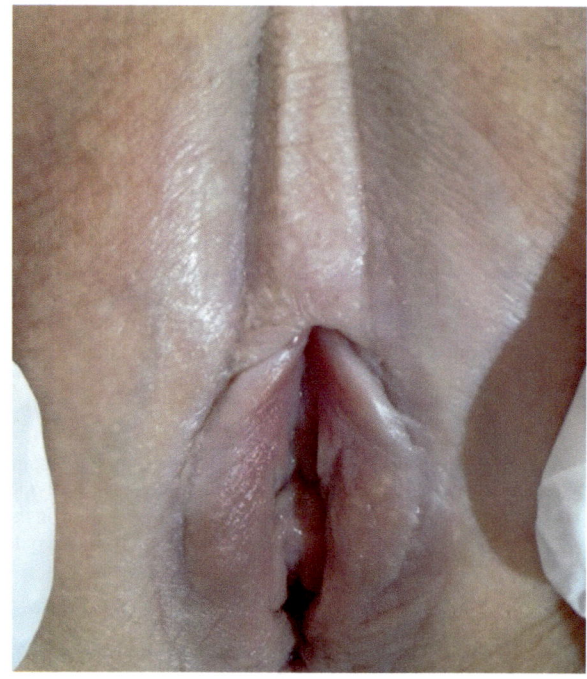

**Fig. 10.1** Vulvar lichen sclerosis (Photo credit: ©Rachel Kornik, MD, 2020). (*In this photo, you can see loss of architecture of the labia with fusion of the labia minora, clitoral hood phimosis, and narrowing of the vagina introitus. The classic thinned, whitened "cigarette paper" skin changes are seen around the clitoris*)

One possible regimen is daily application for 4 weeks, followed by application every other day for 4 weeks, followed by twice-weekly application for 4 weeks. Long-term therapy with either treatment on an as needed basis or with twice-weekly maintenance dosing is reasonable and should be based on individual patient symptoms and treatment side effects. Other treatment options that have been studied with varying degrees of evidence include intralesional corticosteroids injections, retinoids, immune-modulating creams, laser ablation, cryotherapy, and vulvectomy [3, 21]. (See reference [21] for more information on alternative treatments for complicated lichen sclerosis).

Due to the high recurrence rate, surgery is rarely indicated for the treatment of lichen sclerosis. The most common indications for surgical management is treatment of malignancy and release of adhesions for symptom management. There is no standard follow-up protocol; however, initial follow-up in 3 and 6 months to confirm disease stabilization is appropriately followed by visits annually. Close follow-up is essential to monitor for disease progression and malignancy, as approximately 5% of patients will develop vulvar squamous cell carcinoma [3, 20, 21, 23]. Educate the patient on normal vulvar anatomy and the importance of follow-up for persistent or new symptoms or lesions.

The Association for Lichen Sclerosus & Vulval Health has a patient handout about how to perform a vulvar self-exam: http://lichensclerosus.org/wp-content/uploads/2012/09/VHAC-leaf-artwork1.pdf [24].

Other vulvar dermatoses include lichen simplex chronicus and lichen planus.

Lichen simplex chronicus is a chronic vulvar skin disease that occurs secondary to repetitive scratching. Itching is caused by different inciting events including infections, dermatologic diseases, and environmental irritants, such as sweating, heat, and topical products [25]. Most patients present with intense itching that is often worse at night, and temporary relief of symptoms with scratching. The itch-scratch cycle is associated with common exam findings. Signs of early disease include erythematous plaques with exaggerated skin lines and broken pubic hair, while signs of chronic disease include lichenified skin with altered pigmentation and possible ulcers or erosions [3]. A range of representative images can be found here: https://dermnetnz.org/topics/lichen-simplex/ [26]. Lichen simplex is a diagnosis of exclusion and it is important to rule out other causes of vulvar pruritus.

On biopsy, histopathology of lichen simplex chronicus includes elongation and thickening of rete pegs, as well as hyperkeratosis. Treatment is removal of the offending agent and low potency topical steroids.

> **Best Practice**
> Make sure to ask a thorough medical history as 65–75% of patients with lichen simplex chronicus have a history of atopic disease [3].

Lichen planus is a chronic, inflammatory, autoimmune disorder that most commonly affects mucous membranes and skin [27]. Approximately 1% of the population has oral lesions that are often characterized as white, lacy, reticulate areas known as Wickham striae, which can also be found on the vulva [3]. Nearly one quarter of this population has genital disease. Skin lesions can present as purple polygonal papules that can coalesce into pruritic plaques often on the trunk and extremities. However, genital skin lesions are more commonly pink with less defined borders. Erosive lichen planus is the most common clinical variant and causes bright, erythematous, erosive lesions that can cause scarring, loss of labial architecture, and vaginal obliteration (Fig. 10.2). The typical symptoms of vulvovaginal lichen planus are pain and burning. Heavy yellow vaginal discharge is also common [28].

> The common P's of lichen planus: purple, polygonal, pruritus, papules, plaques

**Fig. 10.2** Erosive vulvar lichen planus. (Photo credit: ©Laura Jacques, MD, 2020). (*In this photo, you can see erythematous, erosive lesions at 5:00 and 7:00 with evidence of prior scarring, loss of labial architecture, and vaginal obliteration*)

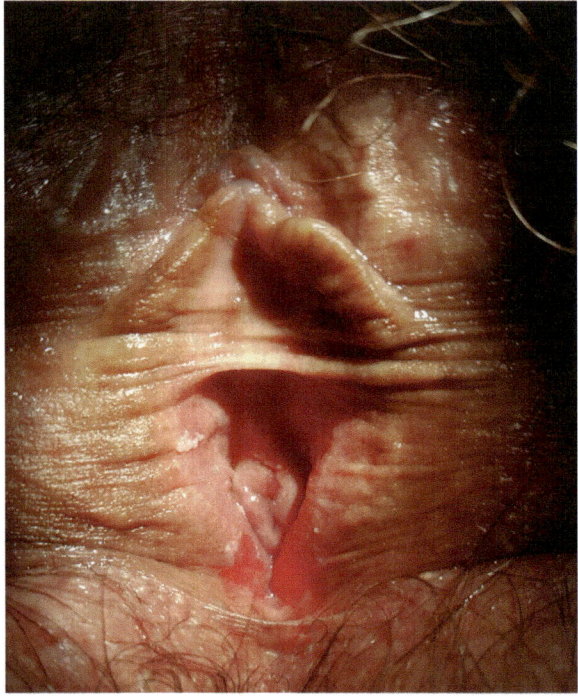

Since lichen planus is a chronic, recurring disease, the goal of treatment is symptom improvement rather than symptom resolution. The most common treatment is daily use of high potency topical steroids that are slowly tapered. Second line therapies include systemic steroids, topical tacrolimus, cyclosporine, oral retinoids, and other immune suppressants [3]. Surgery is limited to adhesive disease and other anatomic complications.

**Best Practice**
Vulvar dermatoses can be complicated to diagnose and treat. Referral to a gynecologist with expertise in vulvar disorders or a vulvar dermatologist is recommended.

**Case (Continued)**
You perform a complete pelvic exam on Carol. You note thinned slightly whitened skin in an hourglass pattern with constriction of the vaginal orifice. Based on these findings you inform Carol that the most likely diagnosis is lichen sclerosis. You discuss the pathophysiology of the disease and treatment recommendations. You prescribe clobetasol propionate 0.05% and make a plan for her to follow-up in 3 months.

**Table 10.5** Classes of corticosteroids commonly used on the vulva [30]

| Steroid class | Examples |
|---|---|
| I: Ultra-potent | Clobetasol propionate 0.05% gel, cream, or ointment<br>Augmented betamethasone dipropionate 0.05% gel or ointment<br>Diflorasone diacetate 0.05% ointment<br>Fluocinonide 0.1% cream<br>Halobetasol propionate 0.05% cream or ointment |
| II. High potency | Amcinonide 0.1% ointment<br>Augmented betamethasone dipropionate 0.05% cream or lotion<br>Betamethasone dipropionate 0.05% ointment<br>Desoximetasone cream or gel or ointment<br>Diflorasone diacetate 0.05% cream<br>Fluocinonide 0.05% cream or gel or ointment<br>Halcinonide 0.1% cream or ointment or solution |
| VI. Low potency | Alclometasone dipropionate 0.05% cream or ointment<br>Desonide 0.05% cream or lotion or ointment<br>Fluocinolone 0.01% cream<br>Hydrocortisone butyrate 0.1% cream |
| VII. Least-potent | Hydrocortisone 1% and 2.5% cream or lotion or ointment |

## How Do You Treat Vulvar Dermatoses? [29]

Vulvar dermatoses are commonly treated with removal of any offending agents and use of topical steroids (Table 10.5).

> **Case (Continued)**
> Carol presents to clinic for her return visit. She notes mild improvement in her symptoms, but continues to report bothersome itching and burning. You recommend another biopsy.

Always biopsy a new vulvar lesion or patients who have persistent or recurrent symptoms despite treatment. You can refer or collaborate with a dermatologist or gynecologist if needed.

> **Best Practice**
> If it's white…take a bite! It is never wrong to biopsy what appears to be lichen sclerosis. Up to 5% of patients diagnosed with lichen sclerosis develop vulvar squamous cell carcinoma! [3, 20, 21, 23]

## Can Vulvar Complaints Be Cancer? [31, 32]

> **ABCDE rule for cancer concern:**
> Asymmetry
> Border irregularity
> Color (change in pigmentation)
> Diameter
> Evolving (in size, shape, or color)

Although Carol's biopsy revealed lichen sclerosis with no evidence of malignancy, it is possible to have cancer of the vulva. Vulvar cancer can occur in the setting of HPV, in patients with lichen sclerosis or chronic inflammatory processes, in patients with vulvar Paget's disease, and in the setting of melanoma (refer to Table 10.6).

- In order to diagnosis cancer, you need a biopsy!
- If a biopsy is negative and there is still high clinical suspicion based on exam findings or persistent symptoms, there should be a low threshold to refer to a specialist for excisional biopsy and treatment.
- If a cancer diagnosis is made, facilitate referral to a gynecologic oncologist.

## What Is Paget Disease? [34]

Paget disease accounts for 2% of vulvar neoplasms [3] and typically occurs in the sixth or seventh decade of life. Exam findings include well-demarcated eczematous, multifocal, lesions with slightly raised edges. Patients typically present with pruritus. A biopsy will show the classic nest of large pale cells with prominent nuclei. Treatment is often surgical with a wide local excision, and there is a very high recurrence rate. Patients should be referred to a gynecologist or gynecologic oncologist for treatment of Paget Disease (Fig. 10.3).

> **Best Practice**
> In patients with vulvar Paget disease, it is prudent to perform a thorough breast, genitourinary, and gastrointestinal exam. Vulvar Paget disease is associated with a 25% chance of neoplastic disease and perianal Paget disease is associated with an 80% chance of underlying colorectal adenocarcinoma [3].

Table 10.6 Precancerous and cancerous vulvar lesions [33]

| | Etiology | Symptoms | Presentation | Diagnosis | Management |
|---|---|---|---|---|---|
| Vulvar intraepithelial neoplasia (VIN) | Premalignant squamous dysplasia that does not breech the basement membrane. Types: usual type VIN (HPV mediated) and differentiated type VIN (non-HPV mediated, associated with chronic inflammatory lesions). Risk factors: HPV, tobacco use, immunosuppression, chronic inflammatory diseases | Asymptomatic, pruritus | Unifocal or multifocal, raised, pigmented, on non-hair bearing areas | Colposcopy and biopsy | Treatment depends on the degree of dysplasia and includes from observation, topical treatment, laser, and excision |
| Vulvar cancer | Accounts for 4–5% of gynecologic cancers. Types: squamous cell carcinoma (>90%), melanoma (~5%), adenocarcinoma, basal cell carcinoma, sarcoma, undifferentiated carcinoma. Risk factors: HPV, tobacco use, immunosuppression | Asymptomatic, pruritus, dysuria, discharge, bleeding | Median age of 68, palpable lump or visible lesion | Biopsy (NOT excision) >50% of patients present with localized disease | Treatment depends on disease stage and includes radical excision, radical vulvectomy with lymph node dissection, and chemoradiation |
| Paget disease | Accounts for 1–2% of vulvar malignancies | Pruritus, visible lesion | Sharply demarcated, pink-red "velvet-like" lesions, more common in white postmenopausal women (see Fig. 10.3) | Biopsy | Wide local excision, active surveillance given high recurrence rate |

**Fig. 10.3** Vulvar Paget disease. (Photo credit: ©Rachel Kornik, MD, 2020) (*In this photo, you can see well-demarcated eczematous, multifocal, lesions with slightly raised edges*)

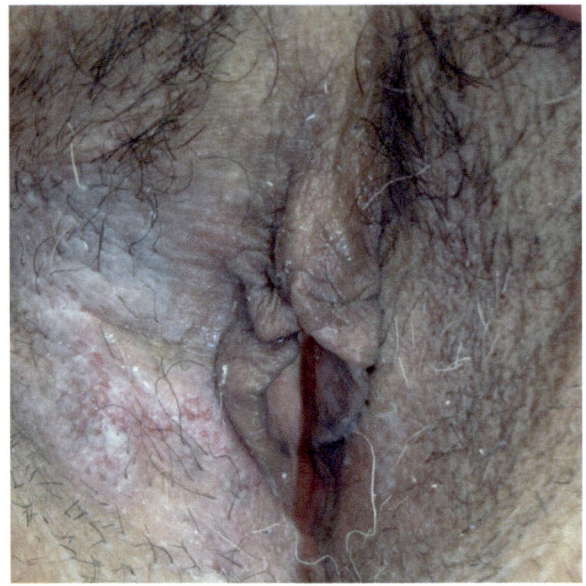

## Wrap-Up

Providers caring for postmenopausal women should be aware of the prevalence of vulvovaginal complaints and the substantial impact it can have on patients' lives. Asking patients if they have symptoms, and performing a thorough physical exam, will help identify women with concerns. Knowledge of the many different causes of vulvovaginal complaints will allow for a supportive patient–provider relationship that provides appropriate treatment and disease surveillance.

## References

1. Hansen A, Carr K, Jensen JT. Characteristics and initial diagnoses in women presenting to a referral center for vulvovaginal disorders in 1996-2000. J Reprod Med. 2002;47(10):854–60.
2. Foster DC. Vulvar disease. Obstet Gynecol. 2002;100(1):145–63.
3. ACOG Practice Bulletin No. 93: diagnosis and management of vulvar skin disorders. Obstet Gynecol. 2008;111(5):1243–53.
4. Johnston SL, Farrell SA, Bouchard C, Beckerson LA, Comeau M, Lefebvre G, et al. The detection and management of vaginal atrophy. J Obstet Gynaecol Can. 2004;26(5):503–15.
5. Summers PR, Hunn J. Unique dermatologic aspects of the postmenopausal vulva. Clin Obstet Gynecol. 2007;50(3):745–51.
6. Fischer GO. The commonest causes of symptomatic vulvar disease: a dermatologist's perspective. Australas J Dermatol. 1996;37(1):12–8.
7. Crone AM, Stewart EJ, Wojnarowska F, Powell SM. Aetiological factors in vulvar dermatitis. J Eur Acad Dermatol Venereol. 2000;14(3):181–6.
8. Farage M, Maibach H. Lifetime changes in the vulva and vagina. Arch Gynecol Obstet. 2006;273(4):195–202.

9. Center SSHPT. Examination of Vaginal Wet Preps. YouTube; 2015. p. https://www.youtube.com/watch?v=8dgeOPGx6YI
10. Paladine HL, Desai UA. Vaginitis: diagnosis and treatment. Am Fam Physician. 2018;97(5):321–9.
11. Paavonen JA, Brunham RC. Vaginitis in nonpregnant patients: ACOG practice bulletin number 215. Obstet Gynecol. 2020;135(5):1229–30.
12. Workowski KA, Berman S, (CDC) CfDCaP. Sexually transmitted diseases treatment guidelines, 2010. MMWR Recomm Rep. 2010;59(RR-12):1–110.
13. Minichiello V, Rahman S, Hawkes G, Pitts M. STI epidemiology in the global older population: emerging challenges. Perspect Public Health. 2012;132(4):178–81.
14. Leiblum S, Bachmann G, Kemmann E, Colburn D, Swartzman L. Vaginal atrophy in the postmenopausal woman. The importance of sexual activity and hormones. JAMA. 1983;249(16):2195–8.
15. Marren P, Wojnarowska F, Powell S. Allergic contact dermatitis and vulvar dermatoses. Br J Dermatol. 1992;126(1):52–6.
16. Margesson LJ. Contact dermatitis of the vulva. Dermatol Ther. 2004;17(1):20–7.
17. Disease ISftSoV. Contact dermatitis of the vulva; 2013.
18. Kingston A. The postmenopausal vulva. Obstet Gynaecol. 2009;11:253–9.
19. Johnson NR, Scheinman PL, Watson AJ. Vulvar dermatitis. UpToDate. UpToDate; 2019.
20. Funaro D. Lichen sclerosus: a review and practical approach. Dermatol Ther. 2004;17(1):28–37.
21. Smith YR, Haefner HK. Vulvar lichen sclerosus: pathophysiology and treatment. Am J Clin Dermatol. 2004;5(2):105–25.
22. Vulvar Biopsy Full Details Procedures Consult2. YouTube; 2017. https://www.youtube.com/watch?v=T3G6RapA7gA
23. Val I, Almeida G. An overview of lichen sclerosus. Clin Obstet Gynecol. 2005;48(4):808–17.
24. Health AfLSV. CLIT: check look inspect touch. 2019.
25. Virgili A, Bacilieri S, Corazza M. Managing vulvar lichen simplex chronicus. J Reprod Med. 2001;46(4):343–6.
26. Oakley A. Lichen simplex. 2014 cited. Available from: https://dermnetnz.org/topics/lichen-simplex/
27. Lewis FM. Vulval lichen planus. Br J Dermatol. 1998;138(4):569–75.
28. Goldstein AT, Metz A. Vulvar lichen planus. Clin Obstet Gynecol. 2005;48(4):818–23.
29. Zellis S, Pincus SH. Treatment of vulvar dermatoses. Semin Dermatol. 1996;15(1):71–6.
30. Ference JD, Last AR. Choosing topical corticosteroids. Am Fam Physician. 2009;79(2):135–40.
31. Edwards L. Pigmented vulvar lesions. Dermatol Ther. 2010;23(5):449–57.
32. Kaufman RH, Gardner HL, Brown D, Beyth Y. Vulvar dystrophies: an evaluation. Am J Obstet Gynecol. 1974;120(3):363–7.
33. Weinberg D, Gomez-Martinez RA. Vulvar cancer. Obstet Gynecol Clin N Am. 2019;46(1):125–35.
34. Parker LP, Parker JR, Bodurka-Bevers D, Deavers M, Bevers MW, Shen-Gunther J, et al. Paget's disease of the vulva: pathology, pattern of involvement, and prognosis. Gynecol Oncol. 2000;77(1):183–9.

# Bladder and Bowel Continence in Older Women

## 11

Heidi W. Brown, Candace Parker-Autry, and Angela L. Sergeant

> **Key Points**
> 1. More than 60% of women aged 65 or older experience bladder and or bowel incontinence, but most do not seek care for their symptoms, despite the existence of effective treatments.
> 2. Dual incontinence, the concomitant presence of urinary incontinence and bowel incontinence, may occur in older women. Self-report is limited due to stigma; therefore, screening for urinary and bowel incontinence and dysfunction is imperative.
> 3. Incontinence symptoms are common in older women, but should not be normalized, and patients should be reassured that non-surgical solutions are first-line and effective.
> 4. Behavioral therapy is first line for treatment of urinary and bowel incontinence, including fluid management with minimization of caffeine intake, dietary optimization for fiber intake, body weight management, physical exercise, and pelvic floor muscle exercises.
> 5. Referral to a pelvic floor physical therapist should be considered for all patients with urinary or bowel incontinence.

---

H. W. Brown (✉) · A. L. Sergeant
Division of Female Pelvic Medicine and Reconstructive Surgery,
Department of Obstetrics and Gynecology, University of Wisconsin School of Medicine and Public Health, Madison, WI, USA
e-mail: hwbrown2@wisc.edu; asergeant@uwhealth.org

C. Parker-Autry
Division of Female Pelvic Health, Department of Urology,
Wake Forest Baptist Health, Winston-Salem, NC, USA
e-mail: cparkera@wakehealth.edu

> 6. Referral to a urogynecologist (for urinary, bowel, or dual incontinence) or female urologist (in the case of urinary incontinence), gastroenterologist or colorectal surgeon (in the case of bowel incontinence) is appropriate when women are impacted by their symptoms physically, socially, financially, or emotionally.
> 7. Additional treatment options for urinary and bowel incontinence include medication, vaginal or anal devices, nerve stimulation, and surgery.

## Introduction

Incontinence has been known as a "geriatric giant" or geriatric syndrome for over 20 years. Majory Warrant warned that "a laissez-faire attitude on the part of medical and nursing personnel to incontinence is quite incompatible with modern methods of treatment and care" in 1946 [1]. Yet, we find ourselves today accepting that urinary incontinence among older women is common and perpetuating to normalize it through the lucrative and self-promoting commercialization of protective garments. Indeed, more than 60% of women aged 65 or older who live independently experience bladder and/or bowel incontinence, with increasing prevalence among institutionalized older adults (Fig. 11.1) [2]. The prevalence of bowel incontinence and dual incontinence (presence of urinary and bowel symptoms concomitantly), is similar in older women and men [3].

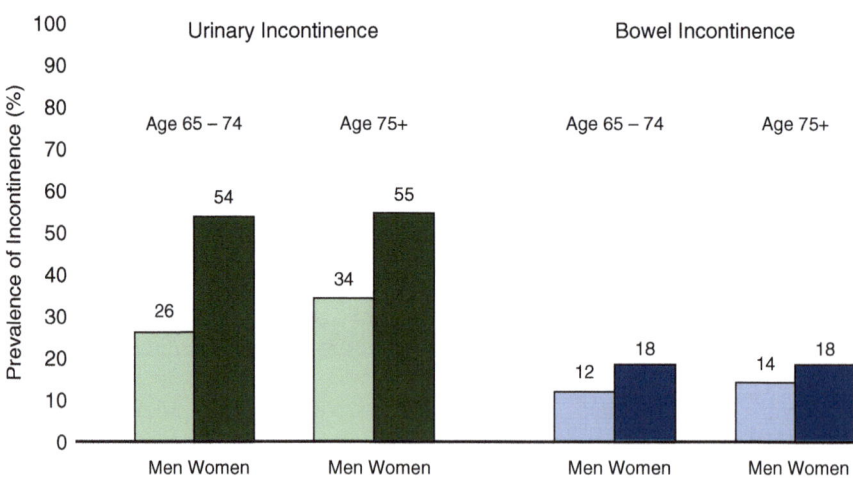

**Fig. 11.1** Prevalence of incontinence among non-institutionalized US adults aged 65 years and older using data from the National Health and Nutrition Examination Survey 2007–2010. (Adapted from [2])

As we age, the significance of vaginal parity diminishes and both bladder and bowel incontinence increase in prevalence even among the nulliparous [4]. This rise in prevalence may be related to the age-related process of sarcopenia where muscle mass is replaced by adipose tissue [5, 6]. There are distinct physiologic changes in the bladder and urethra, potentially driven by estrogen deficiency, which may contribute to this increased incidence of UI symptoms. Though common, the development of UI symptoms is not a normal part of aging. Risk factors for developing UI after the age of 65 years include high body mass index (BMI), functional impairment, impaired mobility, cognitive impairment or dementia, and use of physical restraints [7]. Mixed urinary incontinence is the predominant type, while nocturia, urgency incontinence, and stress urinary incontinence may also be present.

Incontinence increases the risk of depression and social isolation and promotes decreased life-space [8]. This may in turn promote mobility disability and may explain the increased incidence of physical function impairments among older women with urinary incontinence [6, 9]. Both urinary and bowel incontinence can have a dramatic negative impact on quality of life [10–13]. Incontinence is also associated with falls and institutionalization, and is a leading cause for caregiver burnout (Chap. 5) [14–17].

**Case**
Jennifer is a 73-year-old woman with hypertension and diabetes who presents for annual physical examination. She has no complaints. However, during your review of systems, you ask if she has any trouble with losing control of her urine or stool. She starts to cry and tells you that she is "going broke" paying for pads because she has no control of her bladder. She has to rush to the bathroom to void multiple times during the day and night, has uncontrollable loss of urine when she coughs or sneezes, and even when she stands up from sitting. She has completely lost control of her bladder in public so many times that she keeps extra clothes in her car. However, she is now very upset about the onset of trouble with stool leakage that she is often unaware of. Her small bladder pads are not enough anymore. She no longer feels comfortable going out with her friends or to the store due to fear of incontinence.

## The Importance of Screening for Incontinence

Only half of women with urinary incontinence, and fewer than a third of women with bowel incontinence, discuss symptoms with a healthcare provider [11], with a delay of 2 years on average from the onset of symptoms to care-seeking [18, 19]. While clinicians worry that they may offend patients by asking about these symptoms, assuming that patients will bring up these issues if they are bothersome, patients prefer that clinicians initiate this discussion [20, 21]. In fact, screening for urinary incontinence in older women is considered a quality metric by the Centers for Medicare and Medicaid Services (CMS) (Box 11.1).

> **Box 11.1 How to Use Screening for Urinary Incontinence as a Quality Metric**
> The Centers for Medicare and Medicaid Services has a series of Merit-based Incentive Payment System (MIPS) quality metrics (https://qpp.cms.gov/mips/qualitymeasures).
>
> The inclusion of MIPS quality metric #048, "the percentage of female patients aged 65 years and older who were assessed for the presence or absence of urinary incontinence within 12 months," is based on the rationale that many patients will not disclose incontinence symptoms and thus should be asked by a physician about them.

Many patients may not know what the word "incontinence" means, so it is wise to also use simple words, such as leakage, to inquire about symptoms. If your practice includes a written form to elicit review of symptoms, consider including bladder leakage and stool leakage on this form. This form can then open the door for a discussion: "I see you checked off the box about stool leakage. Tell me more about your bowel movements." If you do not use a written form for review of symptoms, using the words "Some people" is a gentle way to start the conversation. "Some women experience leakage of urine or stool as they age. Tell me about your bladder and bowels."

## Evaluation

The initial evaluation of urinary or bowel incontinence symptoms includes a history, including medication review, and physical exam, including abdominal, pelvic, and rectal exam.

## HPI for Urinary Symptoms

In addition to information about the duration, frequency, and severity of symptoms, it is useful to ask about leakage with activity (stress incontinence), leakage with a sense of urgency (urge incontinence), dysuria (pain with urination), frequent night-time voids (nocturia), and problems emptying the bladder (hesitancy, intermittent or slow stream, feeling of incomplete emptying). Asking about the use of pads or absorbent undergarments helps quantify symptoms.

Patients may have bothersome urinary frequency and urgency without incontinence, so an inquiry about number of voids per day and overnight can be helpful.

While voiding frequency depends on fluid intake, a normal number of voids per day is 6–8, with an interval of 2–4 hours between voids. Patients who get up multiple times overnight to void but do not have bothersome urinary frequency during the daytime should be evaluated for sleep apnea. A bladder diary is helpful (https://www.voicesforpfd.org/assets/2/6/Voiding_Diary.pdf).

## HPI for Bowel Symptoms

Even if a woman does not initially disclose bowel incontinence, it is important to ask about her bowel movements and how often she has to strain excessively. A "normal" number of bowel movements per week is between 3 and 20, and gentle Valsalva to initiate a bowel movement is expected. Many patients assume that a daily bowel movement is normal and re-education about the wide range of normal can be helpful.

Bowel urgency, defined as inability to defer defecation beyond 9–15 minutes, is associated with high bother even if it does not result in incontinence. Post-defecation soiling may be a result of incomplete evacuation (perhaps related to stool consistency, posterior vaginal wall prolapse (See also Chapter 9), or muscle dysfunction) or may be related to difficulty cleaning after bowel movements, especially in patients with hemorrhoids or rectal prolapse.

Bowel incontinence is more common with loose or liquid stools and patients should be queried about their usual stool consistency and whether symptoms are worse with certain stool types. Many patients have already identified triggers, such as dairy products, caffeine, alcohol, or spicy foods. Most validated instruments that quantify bowel incontinence severity and bother also ask about use of incontinence products (pads or undergarments), constipating medicines, and impact on usual activities.

Relevant past medical and surgical history should be reviewed for conditions that may contribute to incontinence, including obesity, diabetes, congestive heart failure, constipation, sleep apnea, dementia/cognitive impairment, neurologic disorders, mobility limitations, urinary tract infections, and history of prior surgery for prolapse or incontinence. Vaginal atrophy, also called genitourinary syndrome of menopause (See Section on GSM in Chapter 1), is often associated with urinary complaints, so asking about symptoms of vaginal dryness can be helpful. Women with bowel incontinence should be asked about alarm signs (weight loss, bright red bleeding per rectum, black, tarry stools, night sweats) and whether their colorectal cancer screening is update. Relevant past medical history may include constipation, diarrhea, irritable bowel syndrome, inflammatory bowel syndrome, hemorrhoids, and rectal prolapse, and relevant prior surgeries (cholecystectomy, hemorrhoidectomy, rectal prolapse repair, bowel resection). Certain patients benefit from referral for specialist evaluation (Box 11.2).

> **Box 11.2 When to Refer for Specialist Evaluation (Urogynecologist or Urologist) for Urinary Incontinence**
>
> - Prior surgery for prolapse or incontinence
> - Constant urinary leakage or leakage without sensory awareness
> - Hematuria (at least 3–5 RBCs/high-power field on a urinalysis with microscopy)
> - Recurrent urinary tract infection (2 or more culture-confirmed urinary tract infections in 6 months or 3 or more in 12 months)
> - Elevated post-void residual (>150 mL)
> - Nocturnal enuresis (bedwetting)

## Medication Review

Many medications can contribute to worsening urinary or bowel incontinence. Common classes that can cause urinary or bowel incontinence or retention include the following:
- Alpha adrenergic antagonists for hypertension
- Anticholinergic medications (may cause urinary retention, worsening incontinence)
- Angiotensin-converting enzyme (ACE) inhibitors
- Antihistamines
- Beta-adrenergic agonists
- Cholinergic agonists
- Cholinesterase inhibitors
- Diuretics
- Estrogen therapy (systemic, not local vaginal)
- Insulin and oral hypoglycemic medications
- Muscle relaxants
- Opiate medications
- Over-the-counter allergy medications
- Sedatives and sleep aids

## Physical Exam

It is unusual for physical exam to ascertain a cause for incontinence, but a careful abdominal and bimanual pelvic exam to evaluate for masses should be performed.

Pelvic and rectal exams should be performed in the presence of a chaperone. Visualization of the external genitalia allows an assessment of skin integrity and may reveal changes associated with (GSM, vulvovaginal atrophy) loss of labial architecture and possible urethral caruncle (bright pink tissue lining the urethra protruding through the urethral meatus). Speculum exam is unlikely to reveal a source of incontinence, but if speculum exam is performed, pale vaginal epithelium with loss of rugae also suggests the diagnosis of GSM.

Pelvic organ prolapse may be observed by asking the patient to Valsalva and noting descent of the vaginal tissues or uterus (See also Chapter 9). Pelvic floor strength can be assessed by placing 1 or 2 gloved fingertips gently in the vaginal canal and asking patient to squeeze around your fingers, trying to pull them inward and upward. Copious lubrication should be used. A strong pelvic floor muscle contraction will result in your fingertips being circumferentially squeezed and pulled inward for as long as you ask the patient to hold the squeeze. If a patient pushes outward or downward, performing a Valsalva maneuver instead of contracting her pelvic floor muscles so that the muscles move upward and inward, or if she mounts no contraction or a weak, inconsistent, or brief contraction, she is likely to benefit from referral to pelvic floor muscle therapy. On vaginal exam you may also feel firm stool in the rectum, suggesting constipation may be present.

A rectal exam should be performed in the presence of alarm symptoms or if the patient is experiencing bowel incontinence or difficulty defecating. External hemorrhoids should be noted, as they can make cleaning up after bowel movements challenging and can be the source of post-defecation soiling. Gentle Valsalva while a patient is supine may not reveal rectal prolapse, so if a patient reports symptoms of a bulge coming through the anus with defecation, you may want to refer her to a colorectal surgeon, who will examine her while she is performing a Valsalva maneuver on a commode. Of note, a colorectal surgeon is the most appropriate referral for rectal prolapse (prolapse of the rectum through the anus), while a urogynecologist or gynecologist is the most appropriate referral for vaginal or uterine prolapse (including rectocele) (See also Chapter 9).

After asking the patient's permission to perform a rectal exam, instruct her to gently bear down while you insert a well-lubricated gloved index finger into the anus. Once your fingertip is in the anus, she can relax. With Valsalva, her external anal sphincter should relax, making insertion of the finger more comfortable and also allowing you to assess whether muscle dysfunction may contribute to defecatory dysfunction (if her anal sphincter contracts rather than relaxing during a Valsalva maneuver). Once she is relaxed, you can assess resting (internal anal sphincter) tone, which should feel like a gentle hug all the way around your index finger. You should feel a circumferential tightening of the external anal sphincter around your finger when she is asked to squeeze (like she is trying not to pass gas).

Additional evaluation: A urinalysis is recommended in women with urinary incontinence to rule out infection, glycosuria, and hematuria. As assessment of post-void residual, the amount of urine present after a patient has voided to her perceived completion, should be obtained if you suspect urinary retention. You can evaluate post-void residual using a bladder scanner or straight catheterization. A post-void residual of >150 mL should prompt further evaluation.

For bowel incontinence, colorectal cancer screening is indicated in the presence of alarm signs or if a patient is not up to date on her colorectal cancer screening. Chronic watery diarrhea should be properly evaluated, as should medical causes for constipation, with referral to gastroenterology when appropriate.

**Case (Continued)**
You get more details from Jennifer about her incontinence. She describes worsening urinary incontinence when she started on hydrochlorothiazide for her hypertension. She also says that her fecal incontinence worsened when her dose of metformin was increased to 2,000 mg a day. Her sugars are now well controlled as is her blood pressure. On exam, she has atrophic changes of the external genitalia as well as contact dermatitis from pad use. Her vaginal epithelium is pale with loss of rugae; insertion of a small speculum disrupts the skin integrity at the introitus. Her pelvic floor muscles are tight and tender to deep palpation. You feel a flicker around your fingertips when you instruct her to do a Kegel squeeze or contract the muscles she would use to stop the flow of urine. Rectal exam reveals decreased resting and squeeze tone.

## First-Line Management for Bladder and/or Bowel Incontinence

Initial treatment for an older woman with bladder or bowel incontinence includes education, behavior modifications (Fig. 11.2), and pelvic floor muscle exercises, ideally working with a physical or occupational therapist.

## Education

The patient-facing websites for the American Urogynecologic Society (www.voicesforpfd.org) and the International Urogynecological Association (www.yourpelvicfloor.org) are excellent sources of information for patients, and free written materials can be printed from both of these organizations.

The American Urogynecologic Society offers patient information sheets in both English and Spanish, and has large-print versions available for the most commonly

| Bladder Training | Fluid Management | Constipation Management |
|---|---|---|
| • Schedule voiding every 2-3 hours during the day<br>• If experiencing urge, practice distraction techniques such as deep breathing or counting.<br>• When an urge comes, contract pelvic floor muscles to stop urge. | • Normalize fluid intake; too much fluid results in excessive urine production; too little makes urine concentrated and irritates the bladder<br>• Consider avoiding bladder irritants including caffeine, alcohol, carbonation, artificial sweeteners | • Optimize fiber intake to 21 grams daily by supplementing or increasing intake very gradually and making sure to drink fluids<br>• Osmotic laxatives are safe for daily use<br>• Encourage patients to have a daily plan to manage constipation |

**Fig. 11.2** Behavior modifications to improve continence

> **Box 11.3 Trustworthy Online Resources for Patients**
> - www.voicesforpfd.org
> - www.nafc.org/management-overview
> - www.niddk.nih.gov/health-information/urologic-diseases/bladder-control-problems
> - www.niddk.nih.gov/health-information/digestive-diseases/bowel-control-problems-fecal-incontinence

used patient handouts. The International Urogynecological Association offers patient information sheets in multiple languages.

If you want to keep several high-yield handouts on hand in your office, we recommend these ones:
1. Pelvic Floor Muscle Exercises and Bladder Training
2. Constipation
3. Accidental Bowel Leakage
4. Overview of non-surgical treatments for bladder problems

For audiovisual learners, or patients who have difficulty reading, the American Urogynecologic Society also has a series of educational videos.

Many older women access the internet via computer or tablet, so providing a list of trustworthy online resources (Box 11.3) is recommended.

## Behavior Modifications

### Fluids

The Institute of Medicine recommends that women over age 65 consume 84 ounces of fluid daily. Many women with incontinence restrict their fluid intake, which can lead to constipation and concentrated urine, both of which can worsen incontinence symptoms. Thirst decreases with age, so drinking to thirst will not provide adequate fluid intake for most women. Women should be advised to gradually increase their fluid intake and to space that intake throughout the day: drink an extra half-glass of water at breakfast, lunch, and dinner for 1 week, and then increase to a full glass of water at each of those times. Women who drink an excessive amount of fluid are rare over age 60, but those who drink >100 ounces of fluid daily and are bothered by urinary frequency should be counseled to gradually decrease their fluid intake.

Caffeine can worsen both stress and urge incontinence and so patients may try reducing caffeine intake to see whether it improves symptoms. Other fluids that can be associated with urinary urgency include alcohol, carbonated beverages, and drinks with artificial sweeteners. Patients can try gradually replacing caffeinated coffee with decaffeinated coffee and replacing black teas with decaffeinated herbal teas to improve symptoms.

Patients bothered by nocturia should try to avoid drinking fluids within 4 hours of bedtime.

## Fiber

Women aged 50 and older should consume 21 g of fiber daily, while the average American adult consumes 11 g daily. Gradually increasing fiber intake will improve evacuation of bowel movements, which will in turn improve urinary incontinence. Women should be instructed to increase fiber intake gradually to avoid bloating and flatulence, and should increase fluid intake concurrently to avoid worsening constipation. Many women assume that their fiber intake is higher than it actually is. The handouts on Constipation and Accidental Bowel Leakage referenced above provide some education about dietary sources high in fiber.

> **Myth Buster**
> Many women assume oatmeal is high in fiber, but a serving of steel-cut oatmeal contains 4 g of fiber, while a serving of high-fiber cereal contains 13 g of fiber! A Fiber One granola bar contains 9 g of fiber.

Fiber supplements should be recommended for women who do not want to change their dietary fiber intake. Psyllium is superior to other fiber supplements for women with fecal incontinence, and is the only fiber supplement that improves stool consistency to help stools clump together [22]. Patients should gradually increase fiber intake, titrating for stools that are easy to hold onto and easy to evacuate.

## Voiding Pattern

Women should be counseled that it is normal to void every 2–4 h while awake, depending on fluid intake. Women who void less frequently and experience incontinence may have improvement in symptoms by voiding more frequently; setting an alarm every 3 h to remind them to void can be helpful. Women who void more frequently should be instructed to gradually space out the time they wait between voids, increasing the time between voids by 15 min each week, so that gradually the bladder becomes comfortable holding more urine. The urge suppression and distraction techniques outlined in the "Pelvic Floor Muscle Exercises and Bladder Training" handout are helpful for these modifications.

## Weight Loss

For women who are overweight or obese, even a 5–10% reduction in body weight can improve incontinence symptoms by 50–70%. The contribution of excess weight to their incontinence symptoms should be discussed using a sensitive and nonjudgmental approach (See also Chapter 7).

## Pelvic Floor Muscle Exercises

While patients may improve from doing pelvic floor muscle exercises, or Kegel squeezes, on their own, these exercises are more effective when they are supervised, meaning when a patient receives instruction from a physical or occupational therapist with pelvic floor training. It is helpful to let patients know that this physical therapy may involve additional internal exams, multiple visits, and prescribed exercises at home up to 2–3 times daily.

You can visit www.apta.org to search for physical therapists in your area, filtering results to identify those with training in incontinence or pelvic floor. This resource is not an exhaustive list. If there are no providers when you filter results, it is worth contacting a general physical therapy group in your area and asking them whether and where professionals with pelvic floor training are available in your area.

If you believe a patient has high pelvic floor tone, doing Kegel exercises will worsen her symptoms, so she should not be counseled to do these exercises on her own. If a patient has low pelvic floor tone, and cannot contract her pelvic floor muscles when you examine her, she is unlikely to see a benefit from doing these exercises by herself at home. Those women who have decreased pelvic floor tone, and who are able to contract their pelvic floor muscles when you examine them, are good candidates for pelvic floor muscle exercises on their own, and you can direct them to the educational resources above.

## Skin Hygiene and Containment Products

The vulva, perineum, and perianal tissues are very sensitive. This skin should be kept clean and dry. Dabbing rather than wiping will minimize skin disruption. Using a thin layer of a barrier cream or ointment such as zinc oxide may be helpful for those patients who develop contact dermatitis. The Continence Products Advisor website is a trustworthy source of information for patients and healthcare providers about incontinence containment products.

> **Case (Continued)**
> You reassure Jennifer that she will most likely be able to improve her symptoms. You start by stopping her HCTZ and putting her on a low dose of Lisinopril instead. You refer her to pelvic floor physical therapy. You change her to the extended release form of metformin, and talk about weight loss as a way to better control both her incontinence and her diabetes, with the hope that you may be able to cut down on the dose of metformin. You offer her treatment for her vaginal atrophy; she opts for non-hormonal moisturizers to start. You suggest that she try to avoid wearing pads when possible and that she use a thin layer of a barrier cream such as zinc oxide to protect her skin while she is implementing these solutions. You schedule a follow up in 2 months. She leaves your office with a smile on her face, feeling hopeful about her future symptoms, and thanks you for talking to her about the incontinence.

## Additional Treatments for Specific Diagnoses and Populations

Additional treatment options vary based on symptoms and may include medication, biofeedback, rectal or vaginal inserts (including pessaries), nerve stimulation therapy, or surgery. The approach to incontinence prevention and treatment for patients with cognitive impairment is different than the approach in patients without memory issues (see Box 11.4).

## Urge Incontinence/Overactive Bladder

Patients with overactive bladder or urge incontinence can follow a step-wise approach to treatment (Fig. 11.3). Following the behavior modifications outlined above, a patient should be offered a trial of medication to improve symptoms. While medication is an important component of the treatment algorithm for urinary incontinence in all women, there is potential increased morbidity of using medications in older women. The majority of FDA-approved medications for urgency urinary incontinence and overactive bladder (Table 11.1) have only modest decrease incontinence episodes (0.3–1.2 episodes) per day [23]. While anticholinergics may have

> **Box 11.4 Patients with Cognitive Impairment**
> - Reminder to void every 2–3 h
> - Constipation management
> - Adequate fluid intake
> - Limiting distance from toilet (consider bedside commode)

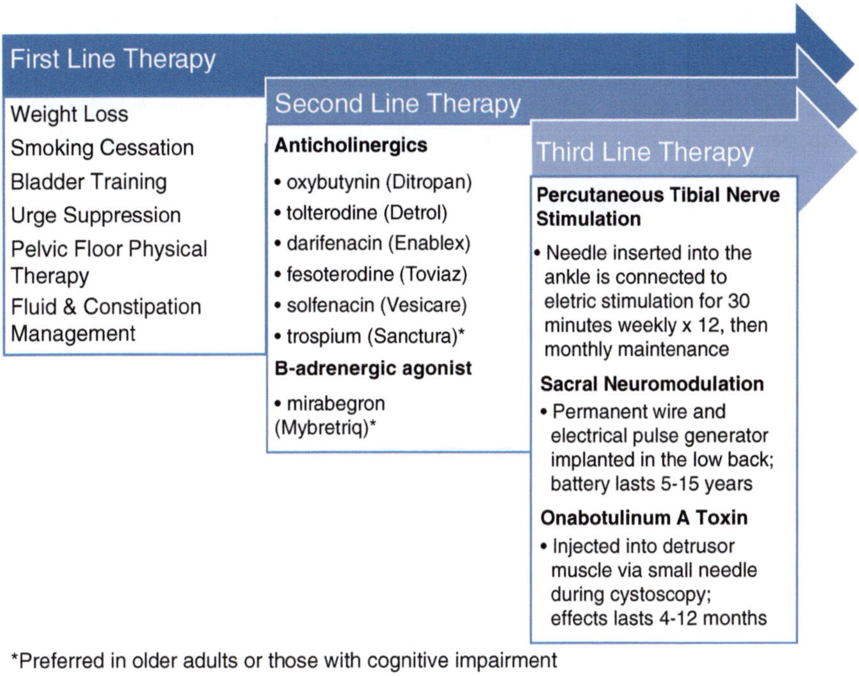

## First Line Therapy
- Weight Loss
- Smoking Cessation
- Bladder Training
- Urge Suppression
- Pelvic Floor Physical Therapy
- Fluid & Constipation Management

## Second Line Therapy

**Anticholinergics**
- oxybutynin (Ditropan)
- tolterodine (Detrol)
- darifenacin (Enablex)
- fesoterodine (Toviaz)
- solfenacin (Vesicare)
- trospium (Sanctura)*

**B-adrenergic agonist**
- mirabegron (Mybretriq)*

## Third Line Therapy

**Percutaneous Tibial Nerve Stimulation**
- Needle inserted into the ankle is connected to eletric stimulation for 30 minutes weekly x 12, then monthly maintenance

**Sacral Neuromodulation**
- Permanent wire and electrical pulse generator implanted in the low back; battery lasts 5-15 years

**Onabotulinum A Toxin**
- Injected into detrusor muscle via small needle during cystoscopy; effects lasts 4-12 months

*Preferred in older adults or those with cognitive impairment

**Fig. 11.3** Therapies for overactive bladder/urge incontinence (Created using information from: American Urological Association and Society for Urodynamics and Female Urology. (2014). *Diagnosis and Treatment of Overactive Bladder (Non-Neurogenic) in Adults: AUA/SUFU Guideline.* * Preferred in older adults or those with cognitive impairment)

**Table 11.1** Anticholinergic medications for OAB

| Anticholinergic medications for OAB | Starting dose |
|---|---|
| Oxybutynin immediate release (IR) | 2.5–5 mg three times daily |
| Oxybutynin extended release (XR) | 5 mg daily |
| Tolterodine (Detrol) | 1–2 mg twice daily |
| Tolterodine (Detrol) long-acting (LA) | 2 mg daily |
| Darifenacin extended release (Enablex) | 7.5 mg daily |
| Fesoterodine (Toviaz) | 4 mg daily |
| Solifenacin (Vesicare) | 5 mg daily |
| Trospium (Sanctura) | 20 mg daily |

a small significant effect on urinary leakage in older women, there is limited evidence to inform its use in the frail elderly, and it should be used with great caution in this population. Common side effects include dry eyes, dry mouth, constipation, urinary retention, and cognitive changes, so we recommend prescribing first for one week to ensure that a patient does not experience bothersome side effects before prescribing for a therapeutic trial (at least 6 weeks). Long-term use and increased impact of anti-cholinergic burden have been shown to increase the risk of cognitive impairment. Trospium is a quaternary amine and theoretically should not cross the blood-brain barrier, so it may be safer in older adults. It is imperative to demonstrate the effectiveness of this medication after initiation through formal assessment of symptoms (for example, comparing number of urinary incontinence episodes or voids per day or night on a baseline bladder diary with a diary completed after 4–6 weeks of therapy. If there is not a significant improvement in symptoms, the patient should not continue the medication. Self-discontinuation due to poor efficacy or bothersome side effects is common.

There are important clinical scenarios in which these medications should not be used, most notably in the presence of narrow-angle glaucoma. Approximately 20–25% of older women have an elevated post-void residual (volume > 150 mL). The mechanism of action of most bladder-targeted anticholinergic medications is to bind to the muscarinic receptors in the bladder to decrease bladder contractility, thereby decreasing urgency and urgency incontinence. In the setting of having a baseline post-void residual volume of >150 mL, it is plausible that use of anticholinergic medications would worsen this condition of incomplete bladder emptying. We recommend monitoring post-void residual once within 4 weeks of starting this medication and discontinuing if post-void residual is >150 mL.

A beta-adrenergic agonist, mirabegron (Myrbetriq), acts by promoting bladder muscle relaxation, and was FDA-approved in 2015. We presume this medication to be safer in patients with existing cognitive impairment. Side effects of the beta-adrenergic agonist can include incomplete bladder emptying and increase in blood pressure. This medication is contraindicated in patients with cardiac arrhythmias but is safe to use in patients with well-controlled hypertension. It is recommended to monitor both blood pressure and post-void residual while on this medication.

It is well within the scope of practice of primary care providers to initiate the first- and second-line treatments for urinary incontinence if they feel comfortable. Women should be referred to urogynecology or urology if symptoms persist. Advanced therapies result in a 60–70% improvement in symptoms for most patients. These therapies include in-office percutaneous tibial nerve stimulation, intradetrusor injection of onabotulinum toxin via cystoscopy, and sacral neuromodulation (an implanted pacemaker to improve bladder and bowel function).

## Stress Incontinence

Following the behavior modifications listed above, women with stress incontinence should consider pelvic floor physical therapy first (Fig. 11.4). Those who are still bothered by symptoms are candidates for an intravaginal device called a pessary or a surgery to improve symptoms, and should be referred to urology or urogynecology for consideration of these options.

An incontinence pessary is a vaginal support device made of silicone that has an additional knob to support the bladder neck and urethra. There are several shapes and sizes available, so fitting is performed by a trained provider; the pessaries used

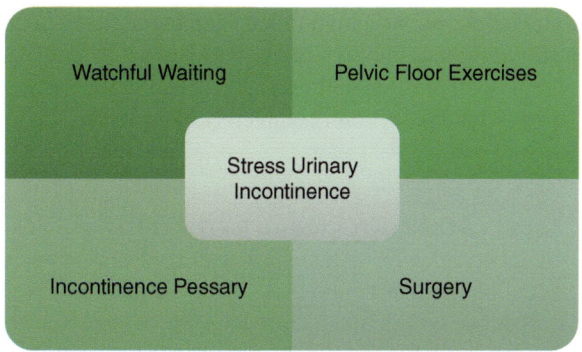

**Fig. 11.4** Therapies for stress urinary incontinence

most commonly to treat incontinence are the incontinence ring and dish. Pessaries can be inserted and removed by a patient herself, or can be managed by a urogynecology, urology, or gynecology office for patients who cannot insert and remove a pessary themselves. Vaginal atrophy should be treated prior to using a pessary to minimize the risk of abrasions to the vaginal tissue.

There are two categories of surgery to improve stress urinary incontinence: slings and urethral bulking procedures. Slings involve placing synthetic or biologic material under the bladder neck or urethra, to keep the urethra closed by preventing excessive movement of the urethra with increased intra-abdominal pressure. Slings are performed as outpatient surgery and have excellent success rates and low complication rates. Urethral bulking procedures are performed in the office or operating room using cystoscopy. Permanent synthetic material is injected into the urethra itself, to keep the urethra closed by narrowing the urethral lumen. Urethral bulking is less effective than a sling, but is also less invasive.

## Bowel Incontinence

Initial treatment of bowel incontinence includes medications to alter stool consistency and delivery and information about hygiene and skin protection, in addition to dietary modifications and pelvic floor muscle training with biofeedback. Intravaginal or rectal inserts and nerve stimulation are also options.

For patients with loose stools or fecal urgency that does not improve with psyllium supplementation, loperamide is helpful. Patients should be instructed to start with half a tablet every other day and should titrate gradually for a goal stool consistency that is easy to hold onto and easy to evacuate. For patients who easily become constipated, liquid loperamide allows for smaller daily doses.

For patients with chronic constipation, a regular regimen to evacuate the rectum will improve bowel continence by increasing the rectum's availability to store stool as it is delivered. An osmotic laxative like milk of magnesia or polyethylene glycol 3350 combined with glycerin suppositories or tap-water enemas is effective for those who are not already laxative dependent. Patients should be queried about toilet height because high toilets, commonly used in geriatric populations, result in positioning that impedes rather than facilitates defecation (Box 11.5). For patients with post-defecation soiling, a 2 L warm tap-water enema after bowel movements will evacuate the rectum completely and may improve symptoms.

> **Box 11.5 Optimal Positioning for Bowel Movements**
> Higher toilets, which are easier to sit down on and stand up from, make defecation more difficult because the pelvic floor muscles do not relax as readily when the knees are below the hips. A step stool or "squatty potty" can be particularly helpful for older patients who need to strain excessively to initiate or complete bowel movements because it raises the knees above the hips, thus relaxing the pelvic floor muscles and aligning the anorectum in a straight line for easy evacuation.
>
>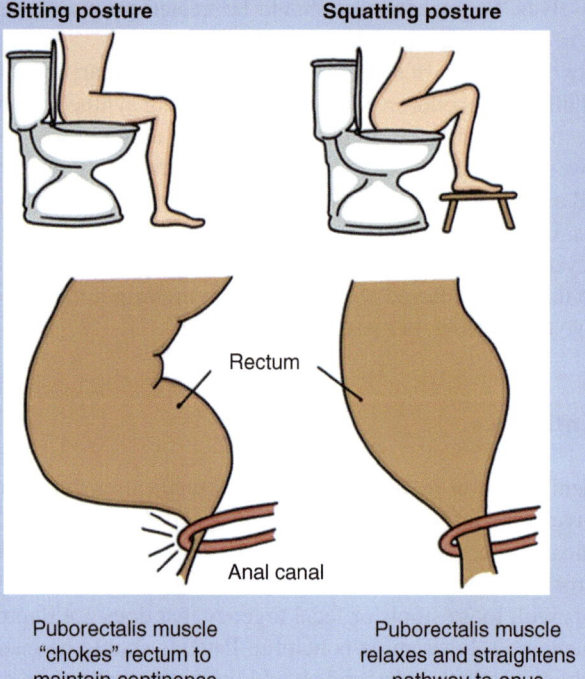
>
> Figure 4.6 Correct posture on the toilet to relax the puborectalis muscle and straighten pathway to anus. (© Association for Continence Advice. CC BY-NC 4.0) [24]

There are several hygiene products specifically for bowel incontinence, including anal inserts, about which more information can be found here. For patients with persistent bothersome bowel incontinence symptoms, referral to a urogynecologist or colorectal surgeon should be considered.

The Eclipse™ vaginal bowel control device is a reusable, removable device placed in the vagina (www.pelvalon.com). Made of silicone, the device contains a balloon that reversibly occludes the rectum when it is inflated. The device is fitted by a trained urogynecologist or colorectal surgeon in the office. The patient wears a trial device for 2 weeks to ensure that it improves her symptoms and that she can manage the device, which requires inflation of the balloon 3–4 times daily and deflation to have a bowel movement. Balloon inflation and deflation happens with a small discreet pump that fits in a purse. For a patient to use this therapy, she must be able to insert and remove the device independently and must have the grip strength necessary to inflate and deflate the pump.

Finally, there are minimally invasive procedural options to improve bowel incontinence, such as injection of bulking material into the anal canal in the office and sacral neuromodulation (electrical stimulation of the S3 nerve through an implanted wire and pacemaker done through two outpatient surgeries). Like the vaginal bowel control device, sacral neuromodulation entails a test period to make sure that the therapy actually improves symptoms. More invasive surgical options, including sphincteroplasty, artificial bowel sphincter, and colonic diversion, are considered for patients who exhaust other treatments and desire additional therapy.

## Nocturia

Nocturia is defined as awakening to void two times or greater during the sleep phase. Nocturia increases in a linear fashion to affect more than 50% of older women after the age of 80 years. Nocturia can be more debilitating than daytime urinary incontinence. More than 30% of adults older than 60 years do not obtain the recommended 7–9 h of sleep nightly because of factors such as social distress, improper sleep habits, and sedentary lifestyle [25, 26]. However, awakening from sleep to void is also a common factor for older women with sleep disturbance, so patients should be asked specifically about this symptom. More information about sleep disorders can be found in the chapter in this book about sleep disorders (See also Chapter 8).

Nocturia can present in isolation or with other bladder symptoms. The causes of nocturia can be organized into polyuria (excessive urine output during the day and overnight), nocturnal polyuria (excessive nighttime urine production), overactive bladder (frequent small voids during the day and overnight), and a primary sleep disorder. The first step in the evaluation of nocturia is to assess daytime voiding frequency, fluid intake, sleep habits, and relevant comorbid conditions and medications in the clinical interview.

Nocturnal polyuria refers to excessive nighttime urine production, defined as >20% of the total 24 h urine production in adults under age 65 and >33% of the total 24 h urine production in adults age 65 or older [27].

A bladder diary with fluid intake and urine output recorded over 72 h will help clarify the most likely cause of nocturnal voiding symptoms is determined. In women with polyuria, causes may include excessive fluid consumption (polydipsia), uncontrolled diabetes mellitus or insipidus, hypercalcemia, or drug-induced polyuria (diuretics, selective serotonin uptake inhibitors, calcium channel blockers, tetracycline, or lithium). Women with nocturnal polyuria should be screened for vascular disease, hepatic failure, nephrotic syndrome, and obstructive sleep apnea. Medication modifications should be considered in consultation with a pharmacist.

In women with nocturnal polyuria, peripheral edema on physical exam may indicate nocturnal auto-diuresis. Compression stockings, elevating the lower extremities before bed, and taking a diuretic in the early afternoon to mobilize excess fluid during the waking hours may improve symptoms. Nocturnal polyuria is found in up to 81% of women with obstructive sleep apnea. Referral to sleep medicine or for a home-based sleep study may help in the evaluation of women with nocturnal polyuria or a normal voiding diary with likely sleep disturbance unrelated to bladder or renal function.

Management of nocturia should align with its cause. In general, we recommend modifying fluid intake to decrease input within 4 h of bedtime, especially beverages with caffeine and alcohol. Sleep hygiene is also important (Box 11.6).

A Special Note on Nocturnal Enuresis: This often requires further evaluation by a specialist such as a urogynecologist or a urologist. If someone is sleeping through the night but finding that she is incontinent upon wakening, it may be helpful to set an alarm once during the night to prompt her to get up to void.

---

**Box 11.6 Sleep Hygiene to Improve Nocturia**
- Limit daytime naps to <30 min
- Avoid fluid consumption within 4 h of bedtime
  - Caffeine is a stimulant and may prevent somnolence
  - Alcohol may increase urine output in the latter half of the sleep phase
- Exercise regularly
- Eat dinner more than 2 h prior to bedtime
- Maintain regular exposure to natural light
- Establish a regular and relaxed bedtime routine
- Create a sleep-promoting environment
- Minimize bright or unnatural light for 2 h before bed and while sleeping (e.g. television, cell phone).

## Functional Incontinence

Functional incontinence occurs when there is a physical delay in reaching the toilet to void, typically preceded by urinary urgency. It can be related to physical disability, but most often is related to the concomitant presence of frailty. Cognitive impairment may also result in a version of functional incontinence when affected persons do not recognize the urge to void or have apraxia, forgetting how to use the toilet. Timed voiding (prompted voiding every 2–3 h) is a very helpful approach to treating this type of incontinence in older women to decrease urinary incontinence episodes. Women who live in assisted living facilities or a nursing home setting may need assistance and it can be helpful to provide written orders for staff. For the nighttime hours, suggesting or ordering a bedside commode can help alleviate the fear of making it to the bathroom when awaking from sleep. Use of foley catheter drainage is not recommended as a solution for urinary incontinence in older women even in the presence of cognitive or physical functional impairments.

> **Case (Continued)**
> Jennifer's symptoms are 60% improved when she sees you 2 months later. Her blood pressure and sugars are still controlled with the lisinopril and metformin. She is still working with pelvic floor physical therapy and can't believe how much the exercises have helped. She is working on relaxing her muscles and contracting them too, and she is using much thinner pads, and fewer of them, than she was 2 months ago. Her physical therapist told her it would take up to 5 months to see the full impact of her exercises, so she wants to keep working on them, and see you again in three more months. Right now, she declines referral to urogynecology, but is grateful for the offer and for the knowledge that other solutions are available.

## Conclusion

Issues with bladder and bowel function are increasingly common as we age. Behavior modifications and pelvic floor muscle exercises improve symptoms in many women. Additional effective solutions exist, including supervised pelvic floor muscle therapy, medications, devices, and minimally invasive procedures. It is important to ask about bladder and bowel issues in an open, nonjudgmental way, reassuring patients that their symptoms are common but not normal and that good treatment options are available.

As with discussion of other stigmatized medical conditions (such as obesity, depression, substance use disorders), it is important to approach a discussion about bladder and/or bowel incontinence with sensitivity. Many women who have both bladder and bowel incontinence will verbally disclose bladder but not bowel symptoms, so inquiry via a written form can be particularly helpful. Urinary incontinence is associated with both constipation and bowel incontinence, so all women with urinary incontinence should be asked about bowel symptoms.

Evaluation rarely requires invasive testing. Treatment approaches for older women with urinary incontinence are generally similar to those of younger women. Clinically severe urinary incontinence episodes among older women may be refractory to behavioral modifications. Pelvic floor muscle training is effective for both storage and evacuation disorders and referral should be strongly considered for older women with any bladder and/or bowel symptoms. Medications, devices, office-based procedures, and minimally invasive surgeries are options for those whose symptoms persist following initial conservative recommendations. The use of medications should be carefully considered in frail older women because of their significant side effects and limited proven efficacy in this population. Setting realistic expectations that urinary and bowel incontinence are chronic and will require ongoing maintenance is helpful, and inquiring about symptoms at regular intervals ensures that patients escalate therapy appropriately.

## References

1. Warren MW. Care of the chronic aged sick. Lancet. 1946;1(6406):841–3.
2. Gorina Y, Schappert S, Bercovitz A, Elgaddal N, Kramarow E. Prevalence of incontinence among older Americans. Vital Health Stat. 2014;3(36):1–33.
3. Wu JM, Matthews CA, Vaughan CP, Markland AD. Urinary, fecal, and dual incontinence in older U.S. adults. J Am Geriatr Soc. 2015;63(5):947–53.
4. Al-Mukhtar Othman J, Akervall S, Milsom I, Gyhagen M. Urinary incontinence in nulliparous women aged 25-64 years: a national survey. Am J Obstet Gynecol. 2017;216(2):149 e1–e11.
5. Cruz-Jentoft AJ, Sayer AA. Sarcopenia. Lancet. 2019;393(10191):2636–46.
6. Parker-Autry C, Houston DK, Rushing J, Richter HE, Subak L, Kanaya AM, et al. Characterizing the functional decline of older women with incident urinary incontinence. Obstet Gynecol. 2017;130(5):1025–32.
7. Inouye SK, Studenski S, Tinetti ME, Kuchel GA. Geriatric syndromes: clinical, research, and policy implications of a core geriatric concept. J Am Geriatr Soc. 2007;55(5):780–91.
8. Wheeler TL, Illston JD, Markland AD, Goode PS, Richter HE. Life space assessment in older women undergoing non-surgical treatment for urinary incontinence. Open J Obstet Gynecol. 2014;4(14):809–16.
9. Erekson EA, Ciarleglio MM, Hanissian PD, Strohbehn K, Bynum JP, Fried TR. Functional disability and compromised mobility among older women with urinary incontinence. Female Pelvic Med Reconstr Surg. 2015;21(3):170–5.
10. Avery JC, Stocks NP, Duggan P, Braunack-Mayer AJ, Taylor AW, Goldney RD, et al. Identifying the quality of life effects of urinary incontinence with depression in an Australian population. BMC Urol. 2013;13:11.
11. Brown HW, Wexner SD, Segall MM, Brezoczky KL, Lukacz ES. Quality of life impact in women with accidental bowel leakage. Int J Clin Pract. 2012;66(11):1109–16.
12. Miner PB Jr. Economic and personal impact of fecal and urinary incontinence. Gastroenterology. 2004;126(1 Suppl 1):S8–13.
13. Shaw C. A review of the psychosocial predictors of help-seeking behaviour and impact on quality of life in people with urinary incontinence. J Clin Nurs. 2001;10(1):15–24.

14. Foley AL, Loharuka S, Barrett JA, Mathews R, Williams K, McGrother CW, et al. Association between the Geriatric Giants of urinary incontinence and falls in older people using data from the Leicestershire MRC Incontinence Study. Age Ageing. 2012;41(1):35–40.
15. Tamanini JT, Santos JL, Lebrao ML, Duarte YA, Laurenti R. Association between urinary incontinence in elderly patients and caregiver burden in the city of Sao Paulo/Brazil: Health, Wellbeing, and Ageing Study. Neurourol Urodyn. 2011;30(7):1281–5.
16. Thom DH, Haan MN, Van Den Eeden SK. Medically recognized urinary incontinence and risks of hospitalization, nursing home admission and mortality. Age Ageing. 1997;26(5):367–74.
17. Grover M, Busby-Whitehead J, Palmer MH, Heymen S, Palsson OS, Goode PS, et al. Survey of geriatricians on the effect of fecal incontinence on nursing home referral. J Am Geriatr Soc. 2010;58(6):1058–62.
18. Bharucha AE, Zinsmeister AR, Locke GR, Seide BM, McKeon K, Schleck CD, et al. Prevalence and burden of fecal incontinence: a population-based study in women. Gastroenterology. 2005;129(1):42–9.
19. Johanson JF, Lafferty J. Epidemiology of fecal incontinence: the silent affliction. Am J Gastroenterol. 1996;91(1):33–6.
20. Brown HW, Guan W, Schmuhl NB, Smith PD, Whitehead WE, Rogers RG. If we don't ask, they won't tell: screening for urinary and fecal incontinence by primary care providers. J Am Board Fam Med. 2018;31(5):774–82.
21. Brown HW, Wise ME, Westenberg D, Schmuhl NB, Brezoczky KL, Rogers RG, et al. Validation of an instrument to assess barriers to care-seeking for accidental bowel leakage in women: the BCABL questionnaire. Int Urogynecol J. 2017;28(9):1319–28.
22. Bliss DZ, Savik K, Jung HJ, Whitebird R, Lowry A, Sheng X. Dietary fiber supplementation for fecal incontinence: a randomized clinical trial. Res Nurs Health. 2014;37(5):367–78.
23. Samuelsson E, Odeberg J, Stenzelius K, Molander U, Hammarström M, Franzen K, et al. Effect of pharmacological treatment for urinary incontinence in the elderly and frail elderly: a systematic review. Geriatr Gerontol Int. 2015;15(5):521–34.
24. Association for Continence Advice website (accessed 5/1/2020) https://www.futurelearn.com/courses/understanding-continence-promotion/1/steps/347026.
25. Lee DM, Tetley J. Sleep quality, sleep duration and sexual health among older people: findings from the English Longitudinal Study of Ageing. Arch Gerontol Geriatr. 2019;82:147–54.
26. Léger D, Poursain B, Neubauer D, Uchiyama M. An international survey of sleeping problems in the general population. Curr Med Res Opin. 2008;24(1):307–17.
27. van Kerrebroeck P, Abrams P, Chaikin D, Donovan J, Fonda D, Jackson S, et al. The standardisation of terminology in nocturia: report from the Standardisation Sub-committee of the International Continence Society. Neurourol Urodyn. 2002;21(2):179–83.

# Sexual Health and Function in Menopause and Beyond

# 12

Lauren Verrilli, Madelyn Esposito-Smith, and Makeba Williams

**Key Points**
- Sexual health is important throughout a woman's life, and 65% of women aged 65–74 have sexual encounters 2–3 times per month.
- Female sexual dysfunction (FSD) may impact arousal, desire, orgasm, and pain with sex, and is particularly common around the menopausal transition.
- Common medical comorbidities such as depression and incontinence impact sexual health.
- Having handouts about sexual health displayed in your clinic communicates your willingness to address these issues.
- Providers and patients should identify main areas of concern and brainstorm interventions that can be easily utilized independently.

L. Verrilli (✉)
Division of Reproductive Endocrinology and Infertility, Department of Obstetrics and Gynecology, University of Utah School of Medicine, Salt Lake City, UT, USA
e-mail: lauren.verrilli@hsc.utah.edu

M. Esposito-Smith
Department of Psychiatry, University of Wisconsin Medical Foundation, Madison, WI, USA
e-mail: Madelyn.Esposito-Smith@uwmf.wisc.edu

M. Williams
Division of Academic Specialists in Obstetrics and Gynecology,
Department of Obstetrics and Gynecology, University of Wisconsin School of Medicine and Public Health, Madison, WI, USA
e-mail: Mwilliams28@wisc.edu

© Springer Nature Switzerland AG 2021
H. W. Brown et al. (eds.), *Challenges in Older Women's Health*,
https://doi.org/10.1007/978-3-030-59058-1_12

- Vaginal dryness, also called vulvovaginal atrophy or genitourinary syndrome of menopause, is a common cause of pain and FSD in postmenopausal women.
- Vaginal dryness can be treated with moisturizers, lubricants, vaginal estrogen therapy, and tissue stimulation using massage or vibrators.
- Referrals to pelvic floor physical therapy and psychotherapy should be considered based on presumed causes of FSD.
- Both hormonal and non-hormonal pharmacotherapies may improve certain domains of FSD.

**Case**
Liza is a 58-year-old healthy woman who presents with complaint of decreased interest in and enjoyment of sex. She has been married for 30 years and is monogamous with her husband. Up until a year ago, they had intercourse about once a week. She is now not interested and when they do have intercourse, it is painful.

## Introduction

Sexual function is a complex interaction between biological, psychological, interpersonal and sociocultural factors. Almost half of women (43%) experience female sexual dysfunction (FSD) [1]. This rate increases as women reach the perimenopause and menopausal transition and decreases in women over the age of 65 [1]. Women may experience disorders of sexual desire, interest or arousal, and orgasm, as well as pain. While there are unique diagnoses, such as hypoactive sexual desire disorder, female sexual interest/arousal disorder (FSAD), and female orgasmic disorder, these diagnoses often co-occur and recommended therapies often overlap [2].

*Spontaneous* desire occurs with little to no provocation and *responsive* desire results from direct sexual stimulation (e.g., sexual foreplay, use of erotica). With aging, many women experience a relative decrease in spontaneous desire compared to responsive desire and this shift may cause distress [3–5]. Patients should be informed that this shift is common and physiologic, and be encouraged to discuss and strategize, with a partner when appropriate, ways to modify environmental factors negatively impacting sexual well-being.

The Dual Control Model of Sexual Response (Table 12.1) provides a helpful framework for this evaluation of how to improve sexual function [6]. It incorporates inhibitory and excitatory factors that may impact sexual function and categorizes

**Table 12.1** Graphic Representation of the Dual Control Model of Sexual Response [6]. Inhibitory factors ("STOP") contrast excitatory factors ("GO"), although it is important to note that some factors are repeated in both categories considering individual differences

|  | STOP | GO |
|---|---|---|
| Biological | Chronic pain<br>Pelvic pain or dyspareunia<br>Medication side effects<br>Cancer<br>Neurological disease<br>Urinary incontinence<br>Autoimmune disorders<br>Cardiovascular disease<br>Menopause<br>Hormonal changes<br>Fatigue<br>Addiction | Physical wellness<br>Hormonal changes<br>Exercise<br>Balanced diet |
| Psychological | Stress<br>Low self-esteem<br>Poor body image<br>Depression<br>Sexual trauma<br>Grief and loss<br>Psychological impact from gynecological and breast cancer<br>Anxiety, specifically performance anxiety | Healthy self-esteem and body image<br>Resilience<br>Low stress<br>Low pressure to perform |
| Sociocultural | Religious and cultural values and beliefs<br>Childhood sex attitudes<br>Gender roles and sexual norms<br>Lack of available partner<br>Intimate partner violence<br>Relational conflict with poor communication<br>Partner's sexual dysfunction<br>Hypervigilance from unpredictable or unfamiliar environment | Religious and cultural values and beliefs<br>Childhood sex attitudes<br>Gender roles and sexual norms<br>Communicative and supportive relationship<br>Predictable and comfortable environment |

them as biological, psychological, or sociocultural. The dual control model is analogous to an automobile's accelerating and braking mechanics; the excitatory "GO" factors function as the accelerator and inhibitory "STOP" factors act as the brake. To increase responsive sexual desire, inhibitory factors should be minimized and stimulatory factors optimized.

**Case (Continued)**
Liza describes a strong marriage with good communication. She had two vaginal deliveries and went through menopause at age 54. Over the last 4 years, she has noticed increasing vaginal dryness and difficulty becoming aroused. Her libido has decreased as well. She has no new medical issues and does not take any medications. Her BMI is 27 and she exercises three times a week.

## Obtaining a Sexual Health History

**Feel uncomfortable talking about sex with your patients? You're not alone!**
Many providers experience similar barriers, including our own embarrassment, lack of training, and beliefs that sexual health is not relevant to a patient's chief complaint. The National Institute on Aging has a helpful guide for talking about sensitive issues with older patients. A 2014 article entitled "How to Discuss Sex with Elderly Patients" by Dr. Folashade Omole and colleagues in The Journal of Family Practice offers some practical tips [7].
https://www.ncbi.nlm.nih.gov/pubmed/24905128

Despite a common misperception that sex decreases with age, the majority (65%) of women aged 65 to 74 have sexual encounters two or three times per month [8]. To provide comprehensive care for menopausal and older women, it is important to incorporate questions about sexual health into your routine history, with an eye toward identifying potential factors that could lead to sexual dysfunction and are amenable to intervention [9–11].

Given the limited time in clinical encounters, it may be helpful to start by adding a question about sexual health to your review of systems. More than 50% of menopausal women experience symptoms related to vaginal atrophy, or genitourinary syndrome of menopause, and the majority do not initiate a discussion of these symptoms with a healthcare provider [12], so adding "vaginal dryness" to your review of symptoms for menopausal women is particularly impactful. Simply having educational materials displayed in your clinic or administering relevant screening tools, perhaps at annual well woman exams, can encourage discussion of sexual concerns. The Female Sexual Function Index (FSFI) [13]) is a validated tool that can assess for multiple sexual issues, including low desire and arousal, orgasmic difficulty, and discomfort or pain during sex.

If time allows, the Extended PLISSIT model (Table 12.2), or Ex-PLISSIT [14] offers a helpful framework for assessing sexual health concerns during an office visit, and is appropriate for use with older adults.

**Table 12.2** An outline of the Ex-PLISSIT model [14] with sample questions for each step

| Ex-PLISSIT |
| --- |
| *Ex*: Permission-giving is a component of each step below. |
| *P*ermission: Seek permission to initiate discussion of sexual health and welcome the patient to share concerns. |
|    "Would it be ok if I ask you more about your sexual health?" |
|    "What concerns or questions do you have about sex?" |
|    "Is this concern something that you'd like to further address?" |
| *L*imited *I*nformation: Provide basic and relevant education according to the patient's concerns |
|    "It is common for one partner to have higher sexual desire or different interests." |
|    "Many women continue to have sex regardless of age." |
| *S*pecific *S*uggestions: If the patient is interested, explore potential solutions to address concern |
|    "How do you and your partner talk about your sexual expectations? What would you think about …?" |
|    "Many patients find that exercise improves desire. What are your thoughts on increasing movement during the day?" |
| *I*ntensive *T*herapy: A minority of women will benefit from a referral to a specialist, such as a psychotherapist, sex therapist, or pelvic floor physical therapist. |
|    "It sounds like you've made multiple efforts to improve. What are your thoughts on seeing a therapist who can explore additional options with you?" |
|    "I want to make sure you get the care and support needed to address this concern. If you're open to it, I'd like to recommend a therapist." |

The first step, asking permission, allows the patient to prepare for the sensitive nature of the discussion and welcomes communication of sexual health concerns. Providers should not assume that the patient is knowledgeable about anatomy and function of sexual organs. Limited information can dispel myths and misconceptions. Some patients may benefit from handouts to review on their own after the appointment. The National Institute on Aging has a nice website with information about sexuality in older adults and this information is also available in Spanish. Having handouts displayed in your clinic also communicates your willingness to address sexual health with your patients and may encourage patients to discuss their concerns with you.

Sharing specific suggestions empowers patients to address sexuality concerns outside of their appointments. Providers and patients should identify main areas of concern and brainstorm interventions that can be easily utilized independently. Common suggestions include using self-care to manage stress (e.g., exercise, mindfulness), improving intimacy (e.g., scheduling "date nights" or mornings, for older adults who may have more energy in the morning), maintaining boundaries with family members, and incorporating sexual aids (e.g., vibrators, lubricant).

> **Devices and Older Women**
> Older women outnumber older men, and with age women are more likely to be divorced or widowed [15]. As a result, masturbation is a normal outlet for women who experience desire but are disinterested or unable to have partnered sex. Some women may choose sexual aids such as vibrators or dildos. Women who experience vaginal dryness and/or atrophy might benefit from the use of the Vaginal Renewal Program, which incorporates manual massage and a massaging wand, such as the FeMani.
>
> For more information on the Vaginal Renewal Program, visit https://sexualityresources.com/vaginal-renewal-program

The final step of the PLISSIT model, *I*ntensive *T*herapy, expands the patient's care team. Sexual dysfunction can be exacerbated with age as a result of physiological changes and psychological stressors [16], and can disrupt progress from medical interventions aimed at addressing sexual health concerns [17, 18]. A multidisciplinary approach is often useful to address these psychological and social stressors (box). It is highly recommended that mental health conditions be treated prior to addressing sexual health concerns [19], thus adjunctive referrals to a psychotherapist or sex therapist may be beneficial. Pelvic floor physical therapists are also important members of the sexual health team. A referral to pelvic floor physical therapy is warranted if the patient experiences vulvodynia, vaginismus, constipation, and incontinence. This specialization of physical therapy uses education, behavior modification, and exercises to improve coordination of pelvic floor muscles.

> **Psychological and Social Stressors**
> - Relational discord with a partner (miscommunication, desire discrepancy, infidelity, distrust, intimate partner violence)
> - Partner's sexual dysfunction, such as erectile issues
> - Co-occurring mood disorders or substance use
> - Grief and loss, especially the death of a romantic partner
> - Low self-esteem and poor body image
> - Unclear expectations of sexuality after menopause
> - Sexual shame and reluctance to explore interventions

## Tips for Taking a Sexual Health History

- *DO* use medical terminology when discussing anatomy and sexual practices, rather than slang.
- *DO* be concise and specific during assessment. Rather than using the umbrella term "intercourse," differentiate between oral, anal, and vaginal penetration. Seek clarification if patients are vague in their responses.

- *DO* normalize behaviors and concerns. It can be relieving for patients to know that their problems are normal and can be addressed without judgement. If a patient endorses a risky sexual practice, offer nonjudgmental education that improves safety.
- *DO* use open-ended questions, such as "How would you describe your sexual concerns?" or "What is your understanding of why you experience vulvar pain?"
- *DON'T* assume that the patient is comfortable discussing sexual health with her partner present. Best practice is to offer privacy.
- *DON'T* make assumptions. Ask permission before assessing patients and seek clarification when needed. Be particularly mindful to inquire about the patient's preferred pronouns and use gender-neutral terminology when referring to their partner unless otherwise specified.

### Case (Continued)

Liza's physical examination finds a BP of 125/73 and a BMI of 27.2. The general exam is normal. Her pelvic examination reveals pale, dry vaginal mucosa with a couple of small skin tears. She expresses discomfort with the speculum insertion, but no other abnormalities are noted. Bimanual examination is unremarkable.

## Physical Exam

A targeted physical exam should be performed to identify and inform the patient of normal and abnormal findings that may contribute to sexual dysfunction. The external genitalia should be examined for signs of common conditions that may impact sexual function, including dermatitis, lichen disorders, and vulvovaginal atrophy, also called genitourinary syndrome of menopause (GSM) (See also Chapter 1). At least half of menopausal women experience GSM symptoms that are problematic for sexual intimacy [20], so even slight changes consistent with vaginal atrophy should be noted and discussed with patients. A female chaperone should be present when performing a genitourinary examination [21] and an interpreter, preferably in person, should be available to help communicate the examination and findings if applicable.

Care should be taken to note hypertension and body mass index (BMI) on initial vital signs. Elevated blood pressure, even when treated, is associated with decreased sexual activity in older women [22]. Low BMI may be a marker of malnutrition or frailty, whereas high BMI may be associated with negative body image and increased risk for sexual dysfunction [23].

When examining external genitalia, it is useful to provide the patient with a mirror to follow along in the examination, point out areas of discomfort, and identify relevant anatomy [24]. If a patient has a complaint of vulvar or vaginal pain, vulvar pain mapping can be performed by softly touching various points around the vulva with a cotton swab to determine whether specific areas cause pain [25]. The National Vulvodynia Association has a nice diagram of vulvar anatomy and innervation here: https://www.nva.org/what-is-vulvodynia/vulvar-anatomy/.

The examiner may notice common causes of vulvar pain including contact dermatitis, lichen disorders, malignancies, or pressure ulcers. Lesions that are suspicious for malignancy should be biopsied or referred to gynecology or vulvar dermatology for additional evaluation. Inspection of the perineum and rectum is useful in identifying stool incontinence, scarring, or chronic ulcers that may be contributing to dyspareunia [23].

An internal vaginal exam with a speculum aids in visualization of vaginal walls and the cervix or vaginal cuff. A speculum exam may be particularly useful if a patient is experiencing vaginal pain or irritation but is not required. If performed, it is recommended to use a narrow speculum with lubrication to decrease discomfort from distending the introitus and vaginal sidewalls, which shorten and thin with age.

Sexually active older women with new sexual partners should be screened for sexually transmitted infections. Patients who have undergone a hysterectomy may experience pain at the vaginal cuff, particularly if granulation tissue or exposed suture is present, causing irritation and increased discharge [26]. Abnormal findings on speculum exam should prompt referral to gynecology.

Dysfunction of the pelvic floor muscles, including increased or decreased tone, may contribute to diminished sensation, desire, arousal, and orgasm [27]. A single gloved finger, with copious lubricant, may be gently inserted to ascertain resting tone of the pelvic floor muscles. If gentle palpation of the muscles causes pain rather than pressure, referral for pelvic floor physical therapy to assess for and treat high-tone dysfunction should be considered. Patients with high pelvic floor tone may also have a history of sexual trauma, so screening and referral for psychotherapy should be considered.

> **Case (Continued)**
> You discuss with Liza different treatment options. She can use a vaginal moisturizer and should add a lubricant during vaginal penetration. You also discuss the possibility of using vaginal estrogen for presumed GSM. For her decreased libido, she is not interested in taking medications right now, but would be willing to see a counselor to make sure that she has no underlying depression contributing to her lower libido. She may be interested in talking about medications (i.e., flibanserin) in the future. You arrange for a follow up in 3–4 months.

## Treatment Options

Treatment options for sexual dysfunction depend on your assessment of what diagnoses are contributing to a patient's symptoms, and the approach is often multidisciplinary.

## Psychological Recommendations

Simple psychological interventions can alleviate distress and foster hope when addressing sexual dysfunction in office visits. Regardless of the presenting concern, patients may benefit from normalization, stress reduction, and sensate focus. Building rapport is integral to utilizing these interventions effectively.

### Normalization
Providers should normalize a patient's sexual concerns. Due to the stigma related to sexuality, particularly the role of sexuality in aging, patients may have limited knowledge of which issues are normal or areas of concern. Psychoeducation and sex education should be utilized to correct myths and misconceptions about age-related sexual concerns. For example, the common misconception that sex stops at a certain age may exacerbate psychological distress during menopause and result in dismissal of sexual needs.

### Stress Reduction
Heightened levels of stress and fatigue are correlated with increased reporting of menopausal symptoms [28]. Stress reduction techniques (e.g., mindfulness, meditation, physical activity) should be reviewed with patients to counter the psychological effects of menopause, which may contribute to sexual dysfunction [29]. Mindfulness, a component of meditation, encompasses vigilant awareness of present thoughts, emotions, and sensations [29]. It promotes affect regulation to reduce stress, anxiety, depression, insomnia, and social isolation. Patients may consider incorporating mindfulness into daily activities. One recommendation might be tuning into their five senses (i.e., sight, smell, taste, touch, and hearing) during a regular activity, such as washing their hands or brushing their teeth. Helpful resources include phone apps and literature, such as *The Miracle of Mindfulness: An Introduction to the Practice of Meditation* by Thích Nhất Hạnh and *Guided Mindfulness Meditation: A Complete Guided Mindfulness Meditation Program* by Jon Kabat-Zinn.

### Sensate Focus
Sensate focus (Table 12.3) is a fundamental sex therapy intervention that embodies the principle of shifting from performance to pleasure; it might be helpful should the patient endorse anxiety, pervasive underlying sex beliefs, or low self-esteem. Developed by Masters and Johnson in 1970, sensate focus encompasses *in vivo* desensitization and operant shaping to improve confidence and mindfulness of pleasure. Patients and their partners are instructed to set aside time for massage; however, in this exercise the "giver" focuses on caressing the receiver's body for their own pleasure, rather than tailoring their movement to please the receiver. This intervention is broken down into four stages which can be accommodated according to need and ability. It is important to remind patients that consent can be revoked during this activity if distressed. It is recommended that participants wear comfortable clothing and consider when to schedule this activity and who will initiate. Pleasure is the measure, not performance (e.g., orgasm, erection), and vaginal penetration is an option, not a goal. The stages are as follows.

**Table. 12.3** A brief outline of sensate focus, which is comprised of four distinct stages

| Stage 1 | Alternate physical touch, excluding touch of genitals and breasts |
|---|---|
| Stage 2 | Alternate physical touch, including touch of genitals and breasts |
| Stage 3 | Simultaneous physical touch that can include genitals and breasts |
| Stage 4 | Simultaneous physical touch that can include thrusting and intercourse |

## Stages of Sensate Focus

For more information, visit https://health.cornell.edu/sites/health/files/pdf-library/sensate-focus.pdf

## When to Refer for Psychotherapy?

It is crucial that providers expeditiously refer to mental health treatment if the patient endorses symptoms that cannot be managed within a primary care setting. These symptoms might include chronic suicidal ideation, moderate to severe depression, and posttraumatic stress (See also Chapter 4). One study found that perimenopause is associated with a 35% increased risk of depression, regardless of history with major depressive disorder [30]. Patients with disorders related to arousal or desire may benefit from referral to psychotherapy, couples therapy, or sex therapy. When patients report performance anxiety, depression, sexual trauma, shame, low self-esteem, relational conflict, and environmental barriers, they may benefit from a psychotherapy referral. Patients with disorders related to orgasm may benefit from a sex therapy referral and can be directed to the following resources.

For female orgasmic disorder, consider these additional resources:
- OMGyes: Instructional videos that demonstrate evidence-based techniques to increase pleasure
- Betty Dodson and Carlin Ross: Betty is a PhD Sexologist with over four decades of experience helping women orgasm
- "Becoming Orgasmic" (Heiman and LoPiccolo, 1976)

## Treatments for Sexual Dysfunction Related to Genitourinary Syndrome of Menopause (GSM)

Vaginal lubricants, moisturizers, and dilators are *first-line therapy* to address the many symptoms of GSM. Lubricants are used immediately prior to penetrative vaginal or anal intercourse to decrease pain associated with insertion and friction. Patients may be reluctant to introduce lubricant to their sexual repertoire, so it is important to dispel misconceptions and myths that lubricant use is indicative of sexual dysfunction. Women can feel desire and arousal, yet *not* experience lubrication. Lubricant use is also recommended for all patients with female sexual interest/arousal disorder (FSAD). Local vaginal estrogen is the most effective treatment of underlying GSM symptoms that may be contributing to sexual dysfunction. More information about treating GSM is available in Chap. 1. *Pelvic floor physical therapy* is recommended to reduce pain with vaginal penetration [31, 32]. Focused pelvic floor physical therapy can aid in relaxation of the muscles of the pelvic floor. If vaginismus is suspected, at home vaginal dilators or dilators used under the guidance of pelvic floor physical therapy may be useful. Regular use of vaginal dilators has been found to reduce pain with vaginal penetration by improving vaginal elasticity [33, 34]. The presence of vaginismus should also prompt screening for a history of sexual trauma, with referral to psychotherapy if appropriate. Patients should be counseled regarding the use of vaginal dilators in graduated sizes (either by themselves or with their partner) to promote stretching of vaginal tissues. Vibratory stimulation, applied either to the vagina or directly to the clitoris, has also been studied as a modality to reduce pain with vaginal penetration [35].

## Treatments for Sexual Dysfunction Not Related to Genitourinary Syndrome of Menopause

*Testosterone therapy* may be considered for postmenopausal women with a history of hypoactive sexual desire disorder (HSDD). Absolute testosterone levels decline with age, but as sex hormone binding globulin (SHBG) also decreases in postmenopausal women, there is a relative increase in circulating, or free, testosterone [36]. With the addition of systemic estrogen therapy, SHBG subsequently increases and circulating testosterone levels fall dramatically. Thus, in postmenopausal women, a short course of transdermal testosterone at a dose of 300ug daily may improve desire, arousal, orgasmic function, pleasure, and sexual responsiveness, and may reduce sexual concerns and distress. Long-term safety data and breast cancer risks have not been addressed [37, 38].

Testosterone therapy should only be considered if hypoactive sexual desire disorder (HSDD) persists after addressing all other possible contributing factors, and should include appropriate counseling about its potential risks and unknown long-term effects [39, 40]. Testosterone level should be followed every 3–6 months, and therapy should be discontinued after 6 months if no significant benefit is noted [41]. The safety of long-term testosterone use for sexual dysfunction has not been evaluated; therefore, the smallest dose for the shortest duration is recommended.

Side effects of testosterone, including hirsutism, acne, and clitoral enlargement, may persist even after it is discontinued. While oral testosterone may adversely impact lipid profiles, transdermal therapy has shown no significant adverse effects on lipids, blood glucose, or blood pressure [42]. Limited available short-term data show no impact on breast cancer risk with transdermal testosterone use.

*Systemic dehydroepiandrosterone (DHEA) and DHEA sulfate therapy* are not recommended for the treatment of female sexual dysfunction. DHEA is one of the most abundant sex steroids in women, and is converted to androstenedione, testosterone, and estrogen. Circulating levels of DHEA decrease approximately 2% per year. It has been postulated that increasing circulating levels of DHEA and DHEAS may improve sexual function and well-being, but studies have not shown a consistent correlation between low DHEAS and sexual dysfunction [43], nor an improvement in sexual function with DHEA treatment [44]. Vaginal DHEA suppositories have been approved for the treatment of dyspaerunia.

*Flibanserin* is a serotonin agonist/antagonist which was FDA approved for the treatment of hypoactive sexual desire disorder in premenopausal women in 2015. The SNOWDROP trial was designed to investigate the efficacy of flibanserin in naturally postmenopausal women. Results demonstrated similar findings to the premenopausal group, with modest increase in the number of satisfying sexual events per month, incremental improvements in sexual desire, and decreased distress surrounding hypoactive sexual desire [12], but the drug is still not FDA approved in postmenopausal women. Common side effects with flibanserin include dizziness, nausea and fatigue; patients should be counseled to avoid alcohol consumption within 2 h of its use because of a rare risk of hypotension or syncope when used concurrently [45, 46].

*Bupropion*, a norepinephrine dopamine reuptake inhibitor, has been shown to improve sexual dysfunction when used as an adjunct or alternative to a selective serotonin reuptake inhibitor (SSRI). Treatment with an SSRI may result in secondary sexual dysfunction in anywhere from 30–70% of women [47]. In one trial of women with SSRI-induced sexual dysfunction, participants who received 150 mg of bupropion twice daily reported significantly improvement in sexual functioning following a 12-week period [48]. In some trials, it exhibits preorgasmic effects at a dose of 300–400 mg/day. Of note, it is not FDA approved for the treatment of sexual dysfunction and so this use is off-label.

*Sildenafil citrate* (Viagra) is a phosphodiesterase 5 inhibitor that has been evaluated for the treatment of female arousal disorder. Data from randomized controlled trials in premenopausal women have not demonstrated increased blood flow to the female external genitalia [49]. Sildenafil has not been studied in postmenopausal women and is not recommended in this population.

## Conclusion

Sexual wellness is an important part of overall health in women throughout the life course. Female sexual dysfunction (FSD) is especially common in perimenopausal women and often co-occurs with common comorbidities such as depression, anxiety, incontinence, and thyroid disorders. Effective treatments exist, but many women are reticent to bring up concerns related to sexual health. It is important to inquire about sexual health as part of your routine history; simply having educational materials displayed in your clinic can encourage discussion of sexual concerns. FSD may impact desire, arousal, orgasm, and pain, and recommended therapies often overlap. Treatment is almost always multifactorial, and may include evaluating medical comorbidities, psychological and behavioral interventions, medications, lubricants and moisturizers, devices, and physical therapy. With appropriate treatment, most patients will have significant improvement in sexual function.

## References

1. Shifren JL, Monz BU, Russo PA, Segreti A, Johannes CB. Sexual problems and distress in United States women: prevalence and correlates. Obstet Gynecol. 2008;112(5):970–8.
2. Battle DE. Diagnostic and statistical manual of mental disorders (DSM). Codas. 2013;25(2):191–2.
3. Basson R. Rethinking low sexual desire in women. BJOG. 2002;109(4):357–63.
4. Cain VS, Johannes CB, Avis NE, Mohr B, Schocken M, Skurnick J, et al. Sexual functioning and practices in a multi-ethnic study of midlife women: baseline results from SWAN. J Sex Res. 2003;40(3):266–76.
5. Dennerstein L, Randolph J, Taffe J, Dudley E, Burger H. Hormones, mood, sexuality, and the menopausal transition. Fertil Steril. 2002;77(Suppl 4):S42–8.
6. Janssen E, Bancroft J. The dual control model: the role of sexual inhibition & excitation in sexual arousal and behavior. The Psychophysiology of Sex. 2007;15:197–222.
7. Omole F, Fresh EM, Sow C, Lin J, Taiwo B, Nichols M. How to discuss sex with elderly patients. J Fam Pract. 2014;63(4):E1–4.
8. Waite LJ, Laumann EO, Das A, Schumm LP. Sexuality: measures of partnerships, practices, attitudes, and problems in the National Social Life, Health, and Aging Study. J Gerontol B Psychol Sci Soc Sci. 2009;64(Suppl 1):i56–66.
9. Krakowsky Y, Grober ED. A practical guide to female sexual dysfunction: an evidence-based review for physicians in Canada. Can Urol Assoc J. 2018;12(6):211–6.
10. Maurice WL, Bowman MA. Sexual medicine in primary care. St. Louis: Mosby, Inc.; 1999.
11. Wimberly YH, Hogben M, Moore-Ruffin J, Moore SE, Fry-Johnson Y. Sexual history-taking among primary care physicians. J Natl Med Assoc. 2006;98(12):1924–9.
12. Simon JA, Kingsberg SA, Shumel B, Hanes V, Garcia M Jr, Sand M. Efficacy and safety of flibanserin in postmenopausal women with hypoactive sexual desire disorder: results of the SNOWDROP trial. Menopause. 2014;21(6):633–40.
13. Rosen R, Brown C, Heiman J, Leiblum S, Meston C, Shabsigh R, et al. The female sexual function index (FSFI): a multidimensional self-report instrument for the assessment of female sexual function. J Sex Marital Ther. 2000;26(2):191–208.
14. Taylor B, Davis S. Using the extended PLISSIT model to address sexual healthcare needs. Nurs Stand. 2006;21(11):35–40.
15. Lamont J, Contributing Authors. Female sexual health consensus clinical guidelines. J Obstet Gynaecol Can. 2012;34(8):769–75.

16. Nazarpour S, Simbar M, Tehrani FR. Factors affecting sexual function in menopause: a review article. Taiwan J Obstet Gynecol. 2016;55(4):480–7.
17. Foley S. Biophyschosocial assessment and treatment of sexual problems in older age. Curr Sex Health Rep. 2015;7:80–8.
18. Freeman EW. Associations of depression with the transition to menopause. Menopause. 2010;17(4):823–7.
19. Wincze JP, Weisberg RB. Sexual dysfunction: a guide for assessment and treatment. 3rd ed. New York: Guilford; 2015.
20. Kingsberg SA, Wysocki S, Magnus L, Krychman ML. Vulvar and vaginal atrophy in postmenopausal women: findings from the REVIVE (REal Women's VIews of treatment options for menopausal vaginal ChangEs) survey. J Sex Med. 2013;10(7):1790–9.
21. Committee on Ethics, American College of Obstetricians and Gynecologists. ACOG Committee opinion no. 373: sexual misconduct. Obstet Gynecol. 2007;110(2 Pt 1):441–4.
22. Spatz ES, Canavan ME, Desai MM, Krumholz HM, Lindau ST. Sexual activity and function among middle-aged and older men and women with hypertension. J Hypertens. 2013;31(6):1096–105.
23. Lindau ST, Abramsohn EM, Baron SR, Florendo J, Haefner HK, Jhingran A, et al. Physical examination of the female cancer patient with sexual concerns: what oncologists and patients should expect from consultation with a specialist. CA Cancer J Clin. 2016;66(3):241–63.
24. Howard HS. Sexual adjustment counseling for women with chronic pelvic pain. J Obstet Gynecol Neonatal Nurs. 2012;41(5):692–702.
25. ACOG Committee on Gynecologic Practice. ACOG Committee Opinion: Number 345, October 2006: vulvodynia. Obstet Gynecol. 2006;108(4):1049–52.
26. Dragisic KG, Milad MP. Sexual functioning and patient expectations of sexual functioning after hysterectomy. Am J Obstet Gynecol. 2004;190(5):1416–8.
27. Omodei MS, Marques Gomes Delmanto LR, Carvalho-Pessoa E, Schmitt EB, Nahas GP, Petri Nahas EA. Association Between Pelvic Floor Muscle Strength and Sexual Function in Postmenopausal Women. J Sex Med. 2019;16(12):1938–46.
28. Taylor-Swanson L, Wong AE, Pincus D, Butner JE, Hahn-Holbrook J, Koithan M, et al. The dynamics of stress and fatigue across menopause: attractors, coupling, and resilience. Menopause. 2018;25(4):380–90.
29. Chételat G, Lutz A, Arenaza-Urquijo E, Collette F, Klimecki O, Marchant N. Why could meditation practice help promote mental health and well-being in aging? Alzheimers Res Ther. 2018;10(1):57.
30. Mulhall S, Andel R, Anstey KJ. Variation in symptoms of depression and anxiety in midlife women by menopausal status. Maturitas. 2018;108:7–12.
31. Faubion SS, Shuster LT, Bharucha AE. Recognition and management of nonrelaxing pelvic floor dysfunction. Mayo Clin Proc. 2012;87(2):187–93.
32. Capobianco G, Donolo E, Borghero G, Dessole F, Cherchi PL, Dessole S. Effects of intravaginal estriol and pelvic floor rehabilitation on urogenital aging in postmenopausal women. Arch Gynecol Obstet. 2012;285(2):397–403.
33. The 2017 hormone therapy position statement of The North American Menopause Society. Menopause. 2018;25(11):1362–87.
34. Stinesen Kollberg K, Waldenström AC, Bergmark K, Dunberger G, Rossander A, Wilderäng U, et al. Reduced vaginal elasticity, reduced lubrication, and deep and superficial dyspareunia in irradiated gynecological cancer survivors. Acta Oncol. 2015;54(5):772–9.
35. Schroder M, Mell LK, Hurteau JA, Collins YC, Rotmensch J, Waggoner SE, et al. Clitoral therapy device for treatment of sexual dysfunction in irradiated cervical cancer patients. Int J Radiat Oncol Biol Phys. 2005;61(4):1078–86.
36. Davison SL, Bell R, Donath S, Montalto JG, Davis SR. Androgen levels in adult females: changes with age, menopause, and oophorectomy. J Clin Endocrinol Metab. 2005;90(7):3847–53.
37. Committee on Practice B-G. ACOG Practice Bulletin No. 126: Management of gynecologic issues in women with breast cancer. Obstet Gynecol. 2012;119(3):666–82.

38. Davis SR, Moreau M, Kroll R, Bouchard C, Panay N, Gass M, et al. Testosterone for low libido in postmenopausal women not taking estrogen. N Engl J Med. 2008;359(19):2005–17.
39. Female sexual dysfunction: ACOG practice bulletin clinical management guidelines for obstetrician-gynecologists, Number 213. Obstet Gynecol. 2019;134(1):e1–18.
40. Davis SR, Baber R, Panay N, Bitzer J, Perez SC, Islam RM, et al. Global consensus position statement on the use of testosterone therapy for women. J Clin Endocrinol Metab. 2019;104(10):4660–6.
41. Wierman ME, Arlt W, Basson R, Davis SR, Miller KK, Murad MH, et al. Androgen therapy in women: a reappraisal: an Endocrine Society clinical practice guideline. J Clin Endocrinol Metab. 2014;99(10):3489–510.
42. Shifren JL, Davis SR, Moreau M, Waldbaum A, Bouchard C, DeRogatis L, et al. Testosterone patch for the treatment of hypoactive sexual desire disorder in naturally menopausal women: results from the INTIMATE NM1 Study. Menopause. 2006;13(5):770–9.
43. Panjari M, Davis SR. DHEA for postmenopausal women: a review of the evidence. Maturitas. 2010;66(2):172–9.
44. Morales AJ, Nolan JJ, Nelson JC, Yen SS. Effects of replacement dose of dehydroepiandrosterone in men and women of advancing age. J Clin Endocrinol Metab. 1994;78(6):1360–7.
45. Kay GG, Hochadel T, Sicard E, Natarajan KK, Kim NN. Next-day residual effects of flibanserin on simulated driving performance in premenopausal women. Hum Psychopharmacol. 2017;32(4):e2603.
46. Simon JA, Derogatis L, Portman D, Brown L, Yuan J, Kissling R. Flibanserin for hypoactive sexual desire disorder: an open-label safety study. J Sex Med. 2018;15(3):387–95.
47. Werneke U, Northey S, Bhugra D. Antidepressants and sexual dysfunction. Acta Psychiatr Scand. 2006 Dec;114(6):384–97.
48. Safarinejad MR. Reversal of SSRI-induced female sexual dysfunction by adjunctive bupropion in menstruating women: a double-blind, placebo-controlled and randomized study. J Psychopharmacol. 2011;25(3):370–8.
49. Berman JR, Berman LA, Toler SM, Gill J, Haughie S, Sildenafil SG. Safety and efficacy of sildenafil citrate for the treatment of female sexual arousal disorder: a double-blind, placebo controlled study. J Urol. 2003;170(6 Pt 1):2333–8.

# Index

**A**
Actigraphy, 109
Alendronate, 38
Antidepressant medications, 52, 54

**B**
Bacterial vaginosis, 150
Bariatric surgery, 101
Biofeedback, 116
Bladder and bowel continence
  additional treatment options, 174
  behavior modifications, 170
  bowel incontinence, 177–179
  bowel symptoms, 167
  containment products, 173
  education, 170–171
  evaluation, 166–169
  fluids, 171–172
  functional incontinence, 181
  geriatric giant, 164
  medication review, 168
  nocturia, 179, 180
  overactive bladder, 174–176
  overactive bladder/urge incontinence, 175
  physical exam, 168–169
  sarcopenia, 165
  screening for, 165–166
  skin hygiene, 173
  stress incontinence, 176, 177
  voiding pattern, 172
  weight loss, 173
Body mass index (BMI), 92
Bone health
  alcohol consumption, 36
  bisphosphonates, 37–39
  calcitonin, 40
  calcium, 35
  clinical presentation, 29, 30
  definition, 26
  denosumab, 40
  diagnosis, 33
  diet, 34, 35
  duration of therapy, 41
  epidemiology, 26
  estrogen, 40
  exercise, 36
  fall prevention, 36
  osteoporosis, 32
  pathogenesis, 28
  pharmacologic treatment, 37
  prevention, 33, 34
  risk factors, 26, 27
  smoking cessation, 36
  teriparatide, 41
  vitamin D, 35
Bowel incontinence, 177–179
Bowel urgency, 167
Breast cancer, 16
  epidemiology, 16
  estimating, 21
  guidelines, 19, 20
  harms of screening, 18, 19
  individualizing screening, 21, 22
  life expectancy, 20, 21
  screening modalities, 17, 18
Buproprion, 196

**C**
Calcitonin, 40
Cancer survivorship
  cardiac complications, 81
  components of, 69
  CRP, 79
  definition, 68
  diagnosing and evaluating, 91–93
  diagnosis, 71, 72

Cancer survivorship (cont.)
    endocrine therapy, 81, 82
    fatigue in, 75
    fear of cancer recurrence, 75
    impact of healthy lifestyle, 73
    lymphedema, 77
    malabsorption or diarrhea, 78
    monitoring for cancer recurrence, 83
    online resources, 70
    patient-facing information, 70
    peripheral neuropathy, 80
    post-treatment cognitive impairment, 76
    radiation cystitis, 79
    safety and timing of vaccinations, 74
    sexual dysfunction, 76
    significant financial "toxicity", 76
    solid tumors of adult-onset, 68
    survivorship care plans, 72
    symptoms of anxiety and depression, 75
    symptoms, late and long-term effects for, 77
    tamoxifen, 82
    toremifene, 82
    vastly outnumber hematologic malignancies, 69
Caregiver, 61–64
    resources, 65
    self-assessment, 63
    support, 62, 64
Chamomile, 119
Chronic radiation proctitis (CRP), 79
Cognitive behavioral therapy for insomnia (CBT-I), 110
Contact dermatitis, 151, 152

**D**
Depression
    antidepressants, 52, 54, 55
    bereavement, 55
    differential diagnosis, 51
    elderly, 50, 51
    electroconvulsive therapy, 54
    grief, 55–57
    medications, 53, 54
    non-pharmacologic treatment, 51
    older women, 45–47
    pharmacotherapy, 59
    psychotherapy, 58
    risk factors, 48–50
    selective serotonin reuptake inhibitors, 52
    transcranial magnetic stimulation, 54
Diarrhea, 78

**E**
Elder Abuse Suspicion Index, 47
Endocrine therapy, 81, 82
Estrogen, 39

**F**
Female sexual dysfunction (FSD), 186
Flibanserin, 196

**G**
Genitourinary syndrome, 4
Genitourinary syndrome of menopause (GSM), 148, 151, 195

**I**
Ibandronate, 38
Incontinence, 166
Insomnia and sleep disorders
    causes of, 106
    DSM-5 criteria for, 106
    epidemiology, 106
    evaluation, 108, 109
    herbals and supplements for, 118, 119
    medical conditions, 107
    non-pharmacological treatments
        biofeedback, 116
        CBT-I, 110, 111
        CBT-I, components of, 110
        cognitive disputation, 113–114
        education, 111
        follow up, 115
        paradoxical intention, 114
        relaxation techniques, 115
        sample cognitive disputation form, 114
        sleep hygiene instructions, 115
        sleep restriction, 112, 113
        stimulus control, 111, 112
        symptom tracking, 111
    pharmacotherapy treatments, 116–118
    resources for patients, 120
    sleep efficiency, 108
    sleep latency, 108
    sleep quality, 108
    sleep window, 108
    time in bed, 108
    WASO, 108

**L**
Lichen planus, 155, 156
Lichen sclerosis, 152–155

# Index

Life expectancy, 19–22
Long-term adverse effects of, 69
Lymphedema, 77

## M
Magnetic resonance imaging (MRI), 18
Malabsorption, 78
Mammography, 17, 18, 21
Melatonin, 119
Menopause
  estrogen therapy, 3
  etiology, 2
  gabapentin, 7
  genitourinary syndrome of menopause, 8–12
  hormone therapy, 4, 5, 7
  laser therapy, 12, 13
  nonhormonal therapy, 12
  ovarian function, 2
  porogesterone only therapy, 6
  vasomotor symptoms, 2–4, 8
Mirabegron (myrbetriq), 176

## N
Nocturia, 179, 180
Nonhormonal treatment, 13
North American Menopause Society (NAMS), 5

## O
Obesity and aging
  bariatric surgery, 101
  classifying, 92–95
  clinical risks of, 91
  dietary changes, 98
  FDA approved pharmacotherapy, 100
  intensive behavior therapy, 96
  intensive lifestyle interventions, 95–97
  medication reconciliation, 94–95
  pathophysiology of, 89–90
  physical activity, 97
  prevalence of, 88
  SIDEBAR, 97
  treatments, 98–100
Obesity-related comorbidities, 93

## P
Paget disease, 158, 160
Paradoxical anxiety, 115
Paradoxical intention, 114

Pelvic floor physical therapy (PFPT), 134
Pelvic organ prolapse (POP)
  additional tests, 132
  clinical findings
    history, 128–130
    physical exam, 130, 131
  epidemiology, 126
  pathophysiology, 128
  recurrence, 138–139
  risk factors, 127
  treatment for
    concomitant hysterectomy, 138
    conservative management, 133–134
    functional repairs, 137, 138
    obliterative repairs, 136
    pessary, 134–136
    PFPT, 134
    surgical management, 136
    vaginal mesh, 138
Peripheral neuropathy, 80
Pessary, 134–136
Polysomnography, 110
Post-traumatic stress disorder (PTSD), 58

## R
Radiation cystitis, 79
Rapid Eye Movement (REM) sleep, 111
Relaxation techniques, 115
Risedronate, 38

## S
Sacrocolpopexy, 137
Sarcopenia, 89
Screening, 17, 18, 20
Selective estrogen-receptor modulators (SERMs), 11, 40
Self-assessment, 63
Sensate focus, 193, 194
Sexual dysfunction, 76
Sexual health and function
  biological, psychological, or sociocultural, 187
  buproprion, 196
  DHEA sulfate therapy, 196
  Ex-PLISSIT Model, 189
  extended PLISSIT model, 188
  flibanserin, 196
  GSM, 195
  pelvic floor physical therapy, 195
  physical exam, 191, 192
  PLISSIT model, 190
  psychotherapy, 194–195

Sexual health and function (*cont.*)
  sildenafil citrate (Viagra), 196
  testosterone therapy, 195, 196
  treatment options
    normalization, 193
    sensate focus, 193, 194
    stress reduction, 193
  vaginal atrophy, 188
Sildenafil citrate (Viagra), 196
Sleep efficiency (SE), 108
Sleep hygiene instructions, 115
Sleep restriction (SR), 112, 113
Sleep window, 108
Stimulus control (SC), 111–112
Stress urinary incontinence (SUI), 129
Symptom tracking, 111
Systemic dehydroepiandrosterone (DHEA), 196

**T**
Tamoxifen, 82
Teriparatide, 40
Testosterone therapy, 195, 196
Time in bed (TIB), 108
Toremifene, 82
Total sleep time (TST), 108
Transcranial Magnetic Stimulation (TMS), 54
Trichomonas, 150

**U**
United States Preventive Services Task Force (USPSTF), 30, 31

**V**
Vaginal Renewal Program, 190
Vaginal stenosis, 78
Valerian root, 119
Valsalva maneuver, 131
Vasomotor symptoms, 2, 3
Vulvar dermatoses, 153, 157
Vulvar itching, 145
Vulvar symptoms
  cancerous vulvar lesions, 158, 159
  causes of, 147–148
  causes, symptoms, and diagnosis of, 149
  complaints, 146
  contact dermatitis, 151, 152
  GSM, 151
  history, 146
  infections type, 148, 150
  lichen planus, 155, 156
  lichen sclerosis, 152–155
  Paget disease, 158, 160
  vulvar dermatoses, 153, 157
Vulvovaginal atrophy, 168
Vulvovaginal candidiasis, 150

**W**
Wake after sleep onset (WASO), 108

**Z**
Zoledronic acid, 38

GPSR Compliance

The European Union's (EU) General Product Safety Regulation (GPSR) is a set of rules that requires consumer products to be safe and our obligations to ensure this.

If you have any concerns about our products, you can contact us on ProductSafety@springernature.com

In case Publisher is established outside the EU, the EU authorized representative is:

Springer Nature Customer Service Center GmbH
Europaplatz 3
69115 Heidelberg, Germany

**Batch number: 08823208**

Printed by Printforce, the Netherlands